THE Chic Geek's FASHION, GROOMING and STYLE GUIDE FOR MEN

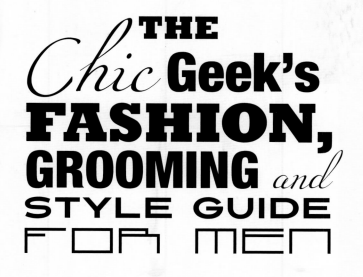

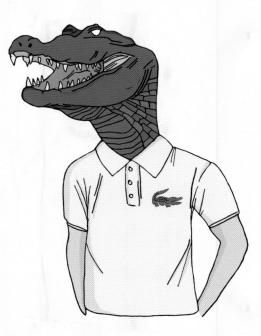

THIS IS A CARLTON BOOK

Published in 2011 by Carlton Books Limited
20 Mortimer Street
London W1T 3JW

10 9 8 7 6 5 4 3 2 1

Design and illustrations copyright © Carlton Books Limited 2011
Text © Marcus Jaye 2011
Foreword © Paul Smith

Illlustrations by Rich Fairhead

A CIP catalogue record for this book is available
from the British Library.

ISBN 978 1 84732 769 7

Printed and bound in China

Senior Executive Editor: Lisa Dyer
Managing Art Director: Lucy Coley
Design: Anna Pow, Barbara Zuñiga
Copy editor: Lara Maiklem
Picture Research: Ben White
Production: Kate Pimm

THE
Chic Geek's
FASHION,
GROOMING *and*
STYLE GUIDE
FOR MEN

Foreword by Paul Smith
Marcus Jaye

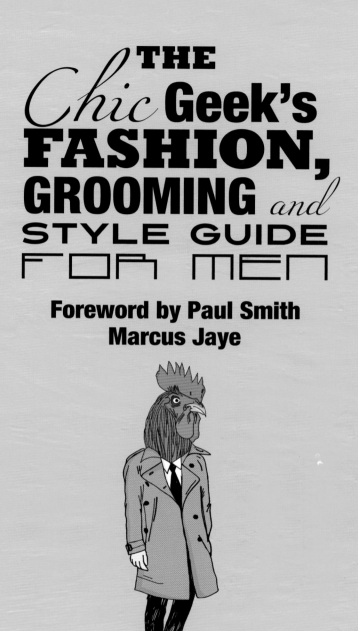

CARLTON
BOOKS

Contents

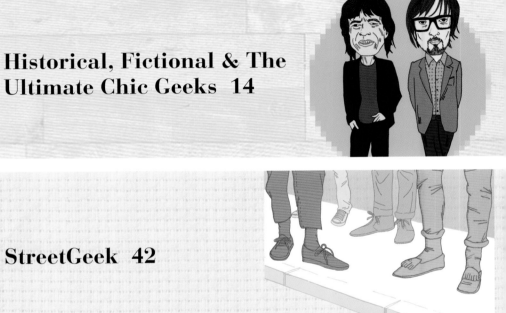

1

Historical, Fictional & The Ultimate Chic Geeks 14

2

StreetGeek 42

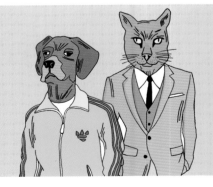

3

Fashion for the Geek 74

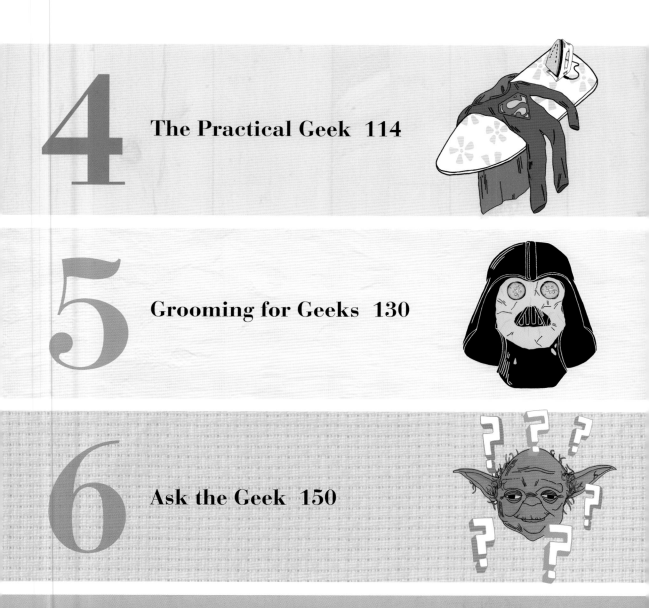

Foreword by Paul Smith

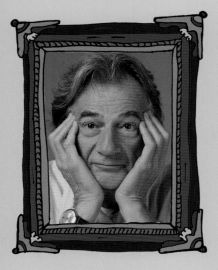

"As a designer with no formal training my influence has always been Britishness, which means to me the love of craftsmanship and tradition mixed with modernity and humour. This could mean taking the influence of a traditional British overcoat but making it in the incorrect fabric or colour or making the traditional coat in the correct fabric but with a vivid printed lining. In other words, always playing with opposites. The other point is taking elements of Britishness; a Harris Tweed jacket for instance and styling it in a way that is unexpected.

Of course the obvious combination from the past would be worn with corduroy trousers and a flannel checked shirt, heavy brogue shoes and a tweed tie. But in today's world it would be a Harris tweed jacket maybe with a denim shirt or washed-out cotton trousers. Again putting together the unexpected or opposite textures; rough and smooth, luxurious and basic. Clothes for men don't change so radically as they do for women and so the attention to detail has always been important because each season as a designer I tend to just nudge my collection from the previous season. This really suits my customers as it is not too radical, more of a evolution. Subtle little geeky details mean a lot to passionate clothes-wearers; real working buttonholes on a cuff, a four-button cuff and always leaving the bottom two undone, or a turn up at the bottom of a trouser just in the right size, 4 cm, mother-of-pearl buttons on a shirt and much, much more. The great thing about stylish dressing is that it does not have to be linked to designer clothes, but it can be a vintage jacket or something found in your father's wardrobe mixed with a designer piece or, in fact, any combinations. Real style comes from within and should be an expression of your personality and also lifestyle and job."

Introduction

Inside every stylish man is a "chic geek". Knowing the minutiae of fashions, materials and labels is what makes a man informed, and hence stylish, and in turn you have to be a bit of a geek to know and care about these things.

Not all men naturally have this, so let me introduce to you The Chic Geek. The Chic Geek is the all-seeing, all-knowing daddy of male style; he's the man we all want to be. He's the best-dressed, most well-groomed, sartorially excellent male and, luckily for us, he's sharing some of his favourite fashion and grooming secrets.

This book strips away the novelty of fashion, leaving behind an underlying guide to male style. It's not about having everyone look the same or conforming to a chosen ideal; it's about empowering the individual, you, to have the confidence to know what suits you best. Style isn't about looking like everybody else but the best version of yourself. There is no point spending time and effort wishing or trying to be something you're not.

Straight-talking and honest, The Chic Geek is always here for all your style questions and dilemmas. As he says, there is never right or wrong, just better or worse. Everything here is a guideline, the idea being to strengthen your judgement in an area that is continually moving and evolving. Under-promise and over-deliver is The Chic Geek's mantra and he hopes you not only learn something but enjoy the process too. Now go make the best of yourself! Enjoy.

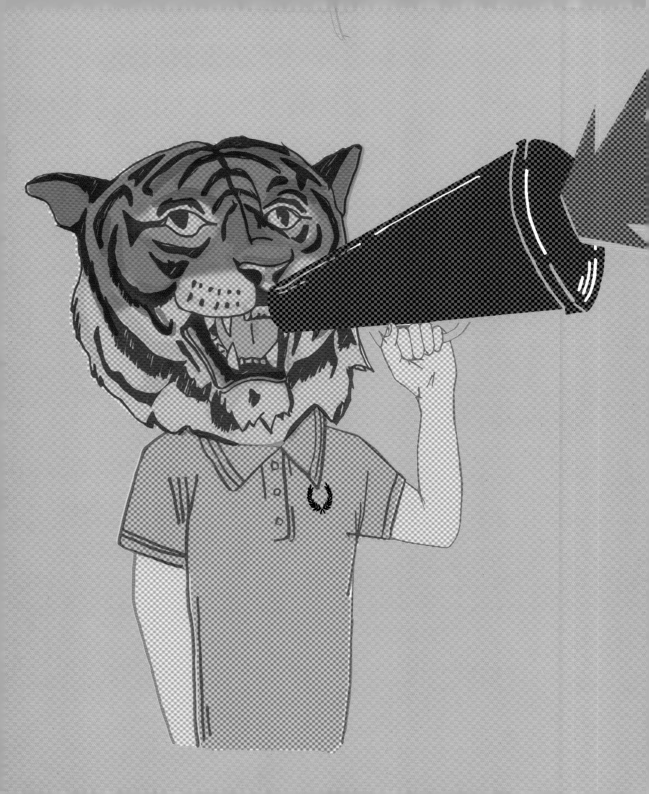

THE CHIC GEEK'S GUIDE TO LOOKING GOOD

One of the first and most important things to remember is that style is not a competition. There is no point in trying to be something you're not because that's not only unattainable but will eventually become frustrating. Work with what you've got and be the best you can with it. If you're short, fat and ugly, then be the best turned-out and attractive short, fat and ugly guy. If you break yourself down to a "type" and strive to be the best, then it's surprising how successful you can be.

There isn't a right or wrong in style. Just better or worse.

Look at other men who have the same characteristics and colouring as you, see what works for them and copy it.

Stay trim and toned. All guys who look good for their age have one thing in common: a lack of belly. From behind they seem younger and from the front they look like a man who takes care of himself. A slimmer frame is far better than any surgery or wrinkle cream for looking younger.

Look natural. Don't hide under too much hair gel, dodgy highlights or the dreaded fake tan. Never overdo it. Consult a professional, seek advice from your hairdresser or from somebody whose style you admire – woman have been doing this for years!

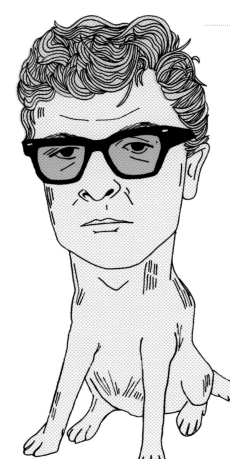

Highlight your best points.
If you have bright eyes, wear complementary-coloured clothing, or if you tan well then wear colours that highlight your bronzed skin. Refer back to point 2 to find out what works.

Be confident.
If you don't feel confident wearing something, then change. If something doesn't make you feel good, take it back or give it away. Confidence is tantamount to looking good.

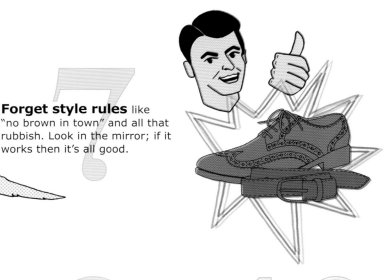

Forget style rules
like "no brown in town" and all that rubbish. Look in the mirror; if it works then it's all good.

Treat your wardrobe like an archive
and keep adding beautiful things. The advice about throwing away anything you haven't worn for a year isn't that straightforward. Some things will come back in time, or might simply be too nice or expensive to chuck out. (It's still good to have the occasional clear out, though, especially of cheaper and seasonal items).

There is a major difference between fashion and style:
fashion is about choice, style is about making the right choice. Fashion is a contemporary list of choices; some years the fashion will suit you, others it won't, so learn what to ignore and what to take on board. Be discerning.

Don't be afraid to look at other guys
and to analyze what you like about what they are wearing and what looks good on them. Remember, certain things will suit some more than others.

11

Sometimes it's not what you wear, it's how you wear it. This often goes hand-in-hand with feeling confident.

12

There aren't two distinct seasons; it's a fashion myth. In most countries we wear the same clothes all year round, so make sure you know your uniform: the jacket that complements your shape, the colours that work and the jeans that make you look good. This is your capsule wardrobe, the skeleton all the frivolous and fun stuff is built upon.

13

Build up your confidence gradually – your style won't be developed in a day.

14

Think retro. Look at vintage pictures of film stars, aristocrats, etc. and adapt their style to look contemporary – the distance of time will allow you to be objective. Some of the most stylish men use this method to look individual, yet rooted in classic style.

15

When you look in the mirror think of yourself as a photograph to be looked at in 20 years' time. Would you cringe? Yes? Then take it off. Things will always look dated, but there's "good" dated and "very bad" dated. You know the pictures I mean!

16

Buy the best you can afford. If you can't afford the best of everything (who can?), then prioritize. Spend the most money on leather goods: shoes, belts and bags. Pay less for T-shirts and knitwear, which, no matter what you buy, often wash badly. An expensive coat is also money well spent; you'll get plenty of wear out of it and it will look good for longer.

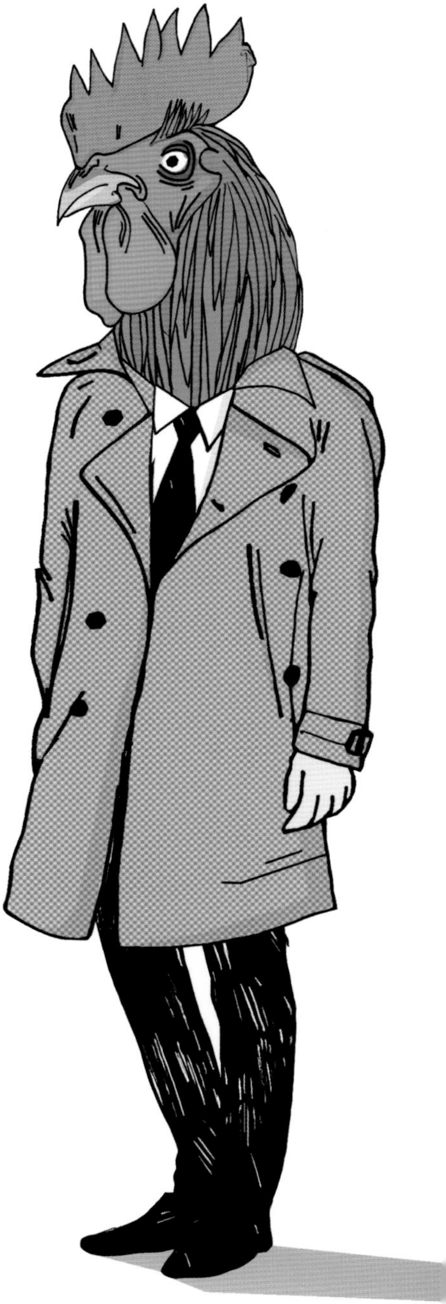

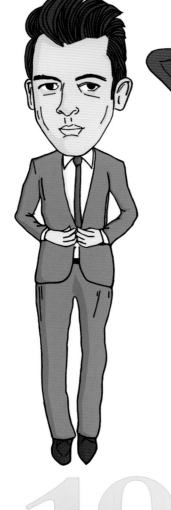

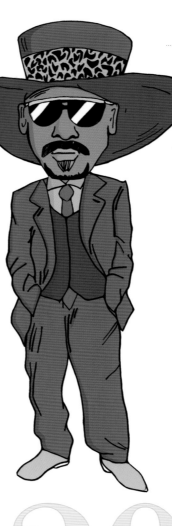

It's all about the fit. You can buy the most expensive item of clothing, but if it doesn't fit properly, it's pointless. A cheap, well-fitting suit is better than a badly-fitting expensive one. Clothes that fit well will also make you feel more confident. Well-fitted clothes can make a skinny guy look larger and a larger one slimmer.

Dress appropriately. Style has changed drastically; where we once worried about being underdressed, we're now concerned about being overdressed. If in doubt, underdress, but not to the extent of wearing jeans to a wedding – there are still some rules about special occasions. Out of respect to the person who has kindly invited you, make some sort of effort.

Don't overdo the frivolous stuff. Too many accessories say "fashion student" and also suggest a lack of discipline and confidence.

Don't wear total looks. A complete designer look that is straight off the catwalk looks wrong, says "no imagination" and suggests you have more money than sense. These days the high street is much improved for fit and choice, so mix it.

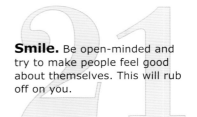

Smile. Be open-minded and try to make people feel good about themselves. This will rub off on you.

Have a break. Indulge in a stubbled Sunday without washing, or do the gardening in an old tracksuit. Just don't let anybody see you!

It might sound strange, but fancy dress parties are a great way to start experimenting with new looks. Before you know it, certain ideas will be creeping into your regular wardrobe.

It takes effort to be stylish. Some might have to work at it harder than others, but inside every stylish man is a chic geek: you just need to be informed and knowledgeable.

Be believable. This means YOU believe it.

Don't be too perfect. Hold a little bit back – don't lay all your cards on the table at once!

Sometimes guys can be so busy trying to be interesting or different that they lose sight of what looks good. Don't be afraid to be objective and step back; less is often more.

Never think you're too cool. Confidence is one thing, but arrogance is quite another and nobody likes a bighead. If somebody pays you a compliment, accept it as graciously as it was given.

Take a risk – looking stylish involves an element of risk. Often the über-stylish flirt with, and sometimes teeter on, the edge of bad taste. It's about touching the line but not crossing it; pushing limits, yet knowing exactly how far you can go.

Don't stress, have fun. None of this is really important life-saving stuff; it's all just a bit of fun and should be treated as such. Enjoy!

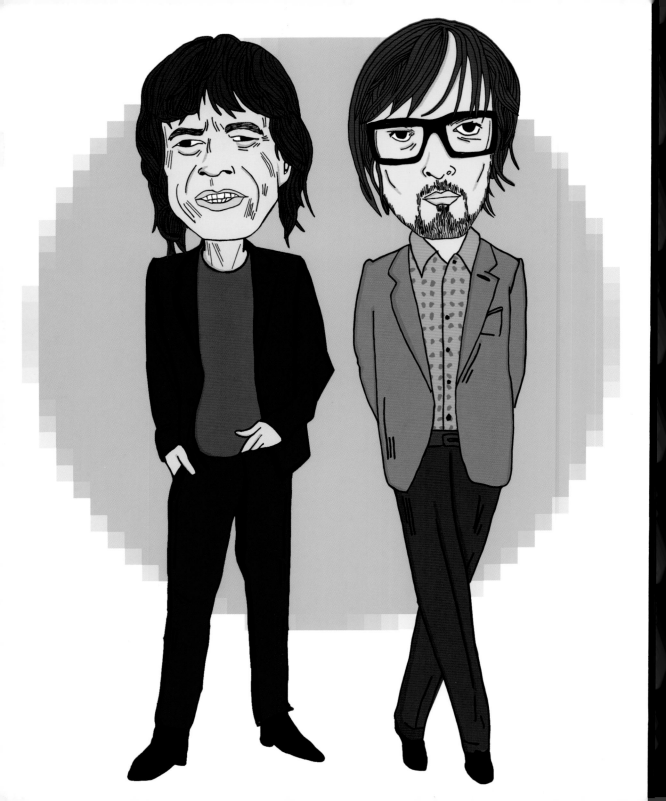

1

Historical, Fictional & The Ultimate Chic Geeks

The Chic Geek is the most stylish man you'll never meet. Nobody has ever seen or met him and nobody ever will. Much like Father Christmas, the Wizard of Oz or even Banksy, you'll only ever see The Chic Geek's work. All his spot-on advice and style decisions are from a sartorially higher place, but he thought it only fair to give you a few famous examples of some mortal chic geeks: men who have entered the history books or our contemporary psyche as the pin-ups of our day. Here is his selection of the all-time favourite historical, fictional and contemporary geeks to provide you with entertaining examples and inspiration when you are getting dressed.

These are the guys or characters that, in The Chic Geek's eyes, have provided an outstanding contribution to menswear or a defining style from their era. This is not about looking good once, it's a continual level of style or finesse; it's about making it into the Male Style "Hall of Fame" and staying there. Royalty, rock stars, movie legends and artists all grace the next few pages. This pantheon of style icons ranges from Henry VIII to Patrick Bateman and every male style god in-between. Start gushing.

HISTORICAL CHIC GEEKS

"Beau" Brummell

Society dandy, George "Beau" Brummell, is the most famous, yet anonymous, man in fashion. A sartorial male myth, his name is well known but his image remains something of an enigma. According to contemporary reports, however, he must have been a sight worth gushing about. Even Lord Byron said, "There are three great men of our age: myself, Napoleon and Brummell. But of we three, the greatest of all is Brummell."

Although Brummell wasn't born into aristocracy he was left a considerable inheritance, which helped him to enter society. Before long his style and wit had gained him access to the inner circle of the Prince Regent. His witty remarks became the talk of London society and he was renowned for his exceptional storytelling and conversation. A man about town, he spent most of his time dressing up, drinking and gambling.

Brummell established the style of understated but fitted, tailored clothes for men that included dark suits, full-length trousers and an elaborately knotted cravat, which became the fashion during the late Georgian period. He claimed to take five hours to dress, changed three times a day and recommended that boots be polished with champagne. "If people turn to look at you on the street, you are not well dressed," he once said. A true metrosexual, Brummell was also fastidious with his hygiene, cleaning his teeth, shaving and bathing daily at a time when it just wasn't the done thing. In her biography of Brummell, Virginia Woolf declared, "Everybody looked overdressed or badly dressed – some indeed, looked positively dirty – beside him."

We have much to thank Brummell for: the suit, the collar and tie, modern trousers and the sombre palette of menswear colours used to this day. He also gave us the humble tape measure and measuring came to be standardized as a result of the "dandy" craze he started. But Brummell got a little too big for his boots when he began to believe his own hype. He went too far when he ridiculed George IV's weight and soon society's doors began to close on him. By this time Brummell was living way beyond his means (we can sympathize!), so when his debts were called in, he fled to France where he died penniless in 1840, aged 61.

Brummell was an exceptional character and had a massive impact on society, which still influences us today. To be remembered as the most stylish man in one of the chicest and most elegant periods of British history really is quite something.

The Bright Young People of the 1920s

Running amok in famous London hotels such as Claridge's and the Ritz, this decadent group of young aristocrats pushed the boundaries of decency and taste. Nicknamed the "Bright Young People" by the *Daily Mail* newspaper, they were Britain's young aristocrats and socialites who epitomized the "Jazz Age" and became known for their lavish parties, dressing up, drug-taking and generally playing around town. Pioneers of the first gossip columns, the tabloids documented their every move, infiltrating parties to report to a fascinated nation.

The brightest male thing was Stephen Tennant (see right, with friends, dressed as eighteenth-century shepherds), an aristocrat known for his decadent lifestyle – it is said he spent most of his life in bed. A 1927 edition of the *Daily Express* described Tennant's headline-making style in this way: "The Honourable Stephen Tennant arrived in an electric brougham wearing a football jersey and earrings." Tennant is widely considered to be the model for Cedric Hampton in Nancy Mitford's novel *Love in a Cold Climate* and one of the inspirations for Lord Sebastian Flyte in Evelyn Waugh's *Brideshead Revisited*.

Documented by photographer Cecil Beaton, this group of creatives and moneyed aristocrats lived life in the fast lane. Among them were names such as the composer William Walton, artist Rex Whistler and poet John Betjeman. They partied in luxe, over-the-top opulence, often dressed in theatrical and gender-blurring fancy dress. This privileged elite entertained themselves in one of the most colourful and briefest periods of history, but like all stars they burnt bright then faded away with the commencement of the Second World War.

The Bright Young People were the first hedonists of the modern age and as such they have given us a romantic image of an overindulgent party type. Mixing society dress and fancy dress, they were not doing it for anyone but themselves, which makes them truly chic.

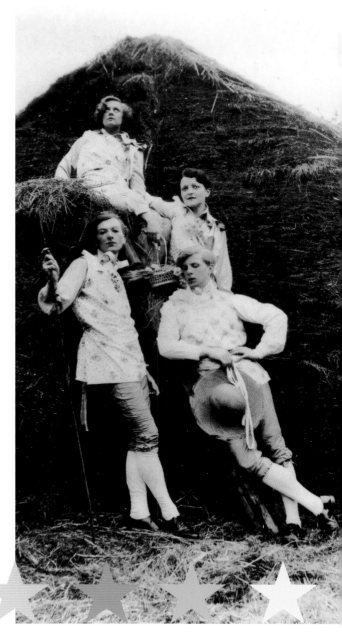

The Duke of Windsor

Formerly Edward VIII, the Duke of Windsor is possibly the most fashionably referenced male of the twentieth century. He abdicated the British throne to marry the American divorcée Wallis Simpson and lived a life of exiled indulgence. Holed up in the Bahamas and France, this Cartier-shopping pair became one of history's chicest couples.

As the Prince of Wales, Edward was well known as a fashion leader – the world looked at what he did and duly copied. He was an innovator of male dress; if he didn't like something he'd change it, and what he did like he often exaggerated. For instance, he disliked braces (suspenders), so he asked for trousers with elastic in the waist; he didn't like buttons on trousers so instead insisted on a zip, which was still large and primitive in the 1930s; he preferred four buttons on the sleeves of his jackets and always wore turn-ups (cuffs) on his trousers; he pioneered a navy bowler hat instead of the traditional black and the famous Glen Urquhart check was renamed the Prince of Wales check in his honour.

The Duke of Windsor was a classic advertisement for Savile Row and wore the same suits in the 1960s that he had had made in the 1920s. This was facilitated by the fact that he managed to keep his figure, which allowed him, with a few alterations, to wear the same clothes for over five decades. This was a man who enjoyed clothes and took care of how he looked. He had fabulous taste – even his dogs (pugs) were chic.

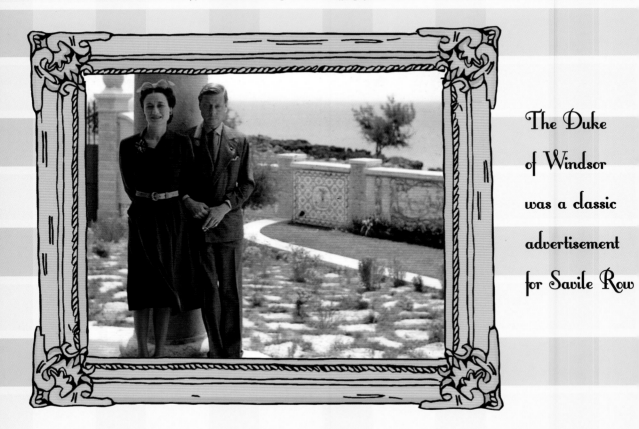

The Duke of Windsor was a classic advertisement for Savile Row

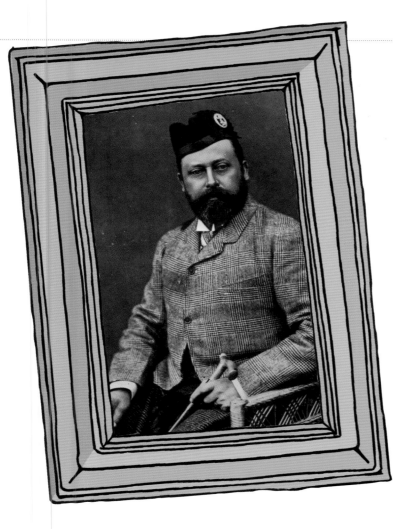

The Windsor knot was actually named after him

uncomfortably hot, so he replaced the heavy "tails" jacket with a short, lightweight version, now universally known as the dinner jacket (or tuxedo). With the development of photography, men were able to keep track of what he was wearing. Everything from his frock coats, light-coloured trousers, smart waistcoats, walking cane, umbrella and light-coloured or white top hats were all copied, creating quite an industry.

We have a number of fashion staples to thank Edward for: the Windsor tie knot was actually named after him, for example, and not the Duke of Windsor. He also pioneered the pressing of trouser legs from side to side in preference to front and back creases and was thought to have introduced the stand-up, turn-down shirt collar. The tradition of men not buttoning the bottom button of suit jackets is linked to Edward, who supposedly left his own undone due to his large girth. Later, Edward inspired the 1950s "Teddy Boy" movement, with young men coping the dandies of the Edwardian era by wearing period drape jackets.

With a full imperial title of "Edward VII, by the Grace of God, of the United Kingdom of Great Britain and Ireland, and of all the British Dominions beyond the Seas, King, Defender of the Faith, Emperor of India", could anyone be more stylish?

Edward VII

Queen Victoria's eldest son, Edward VII, is not often thought of as a style leader, but he was a pioneer of his day. Famous for his sporting, womanizing and leisurely pursuits, he took his wardrobe very seriously, so much so that his puritanical father, Albert, often accused him of dandyism.

As king-in-waiting for a record period, Edward put his spare time to good sartorial use, making tweed Homburg hats and Norfolk jackets fashionable. Once, on a long sea voyage to India in 1875, he found that evening dress was

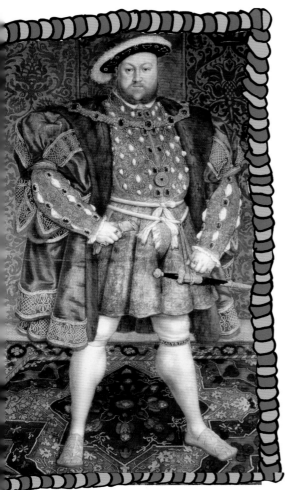

Henry VIII

The last red-haired King of England, Henry VIII wasn't always the fat old bruiser we have come to know. A fashion leader across Europe, as a young man he was said to be very good-looking and his athleticism was well regarded. He was tall with a large and muscular frame, played football and tennis, and liked clothes that showed off his physique. In 1515 an impressed Venetian ambassador wrote, "His Majesty is the handsomest potentate I ever set eyes on; above the usual height, with an extremely fine calf to his leg, his complexion very fair and bright, with auburn hair combed straight and short, in the French fashion."

Henry dressed in colourful clothes, enjoyed wearing jewels, ate and drank well and spent money with abandon. An anonymous foreigner at the time wrote that he was "the best dressed sovereign in the world". When Henry met Charles V of Spain in 1520, he appeared in a "robe entirely of cloth of gold, lined with very beautiful lynx fur".

Henry dressed to flaunt his power, stature and wealth. One of the most famous images of him is the 1537 portrait by Hans Holbein (above), which shows him standing with hands on hips. His protruding codpiece expresses virility and the wealth of fur, pearls and embroidered cloth about his person proclaims his absolute authority. Henry was, without doubt, the best-dressed Tudor male in history... anyone attempting to upstage him would have been sent straight to the Tower!

Louis XIV

An extravagant, absolute monarch, Louis XIV of France was the first king to fully understand the importance of clothes as a symbol of power. The "Sun King", as he became known, was one of the most grotesquely indulgent males of all time, wearing the richest brocades and the finest furs and jewels... he even used lace for toilet paper!

His long reign and wealth put Louis at the forefront of any change in male fashions during the seventeenth century. The wearing of wigs was brought into fashion by Louis, who, not wishing to lose the admiration occasioned by his long, curled locks when he grew bald, adopted the curled wig. He had beautiful long, brown hair in his youth, according to contemporary sources, but became bald early.

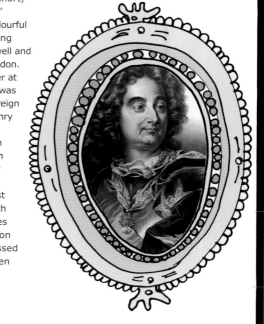

In 1655 Louis appointed 48 royal wigmakers and one year later founded the first Parisian wigmakers guild.

At around 1650 men had stopped wearing the doublet, hose and cloak, fundamentals of a male wardrobe since early in the sixteenth century. Louis XIV is credited with simplifying male dress by authorizing courtiers to adopt the long jacket and fitted breeches that they wore to go hunting, as everyday wear. During his reign men started to wear coats, vests and breeches, which we can recognize as the basic three components of modern attire. Gold cloth was reserved for the Monarch and his favourites at the court and this was regulated by edicts, which prohibited those of a lower station from wearing it.

Sadly few clothes exist from this time, as French royals tended to hand down garments once they went out of fashion to their ladies- and gentlemen-in-waiting. Fashions quickly changed at Versailles and it was a major preoccupation keeping up with them. For this reason Louis XIV makes it onto our list as the world's first male fashion victim.

Oscar Wilde

There are not many guys who are confident enough to wear a sunflower-sized flower in their buttonhole but Oscar Wilde, the Irish playwright, poet and aesthete, was as outlandish in his dress as he was in his prose. He once famously said, "The only way to atone for being occasionally a little overdressed is by being always absolutely over-educated."

Certainly no shrinking violet, Wilde understood the power of image and his attention-grabbing antics complemented his style. He cultivated an "aesthetic lecturing costume" that he wore on his year-long tour of America in 1882. It consisted of long silk stockings, a frilly lace collar, patent leather pumps and a flower (sunflower or lily) that he either carried or wore.

Wilde revelled in the late-Victorian aesthetic movement: think velvet, quilted smoking jackets and knickerbockers. It was reported at the time that he favoured an "open-work embroidered shirt showing a black silk lining, a large yellow silk handkerchief thrust in the breast of the coat, and a high stock [stocking] of the past ages." He had the confidence of his intelligence and wit to know that he could get away with almost anything.

FICTIONAL CHIC GEEKS

Alfie, the Michael Caine version

Alfie is the film of a young predatory male finding out about life and commitment. Michael Caine starred in the original 1966 version and while Jude Law did a good job in the 2004 remake, Caine will forever be Alfie Elkins, the archetypal working-class, cockney wide-boy. Dressed for success, even though he never sticks to one job, Alfie's smart attire complements his gift-of-the-gab way with the ladies. Smart suits (terylene and mohair), skinny ties and a signet ring make Alfie the sobering image of the 1960s. As he says in the film, "What's it all about? You know what I mean."

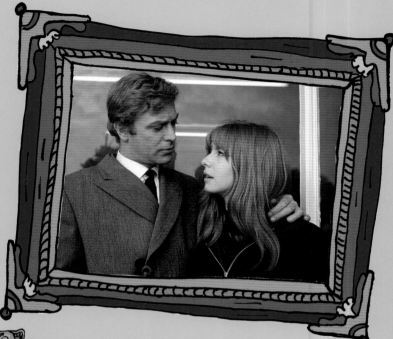

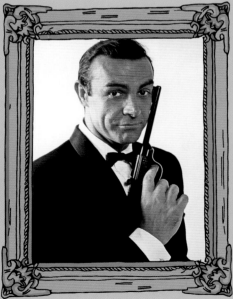

James Bond

007 has had as many looks as actors who have played the part, but his tuxedo has remained constant throughout. From cheesy casino to formal ambassadorial do, Mr Bond oozes evening sophistication like no one else. Created in 1953 by writer Ian Fleming, James Bond featured in 12 novels and two short story collections.

Much like The Chic Geek, Bond is bigger than one man. From the Aston Martin-driving womanizer to the budgie-smuggling beach god, the secret agent's dress sense is never shaken or stirred. In the books his basic outfit is a dark blue suit of serge, tropical worsted or alpaca depending on the climate, a heavy white silk shirt, a thin black knitted silk tie, dark blue socks and well-polished, black moccasin-style shoes. On-screen, Brioni, Tom Ford, Omega, Sunspel and Church's are just some of the exclusive brands to have made up Bond's wardrobe. Definitely somebody on our jetsetting, man-of-mystery list to aspire to.

Patrick Bateman from American Psycho

Perhaps the most stylish serial killer ever. Patrick Bateman is the central character in Bret Easton Ellis's 1991 novel *American Psycho*, which was later turned into a movie starring Christian Bale as Bateman. We love a man this anal about everything, from his clothes and the restaurants he eats in to his business cards. An investment banker, Bateman has the disposable income to indulge his love of labels – Jean Paul Gaultier, Oliver Peoples and Valentino to name just a few – but it is his grooming routine that makes him the ultimate chic geek.

My name is Patrick Bateman. I'm 27 years old. I believe in taking care of myself and a balanced diet and rigorous exercise routine. In the morning if my face is a little puffy I'll put on an ice pack while doing stomach crunches. I can do 1,000 now. After I remove the ice pack I use a deep pore cleanser lotion. In the shower I use a water-activated gel cleanser, then a honey almond body scrub, and on the face an exfoliating gel scrub. Then I apply an herb-mint facial mask, which I leave on for 10 minutes while I prepare the rest of my routine. I always use an aftershave lotion with little or no alcohol, because alcohol dries your face out and makes you look older. Then moisturizer, then an anti-aging eye balm, followed by a final moisturizing protective lotion.

Legend!

Benjamin Braddock from The Graduate

Dustin Hoffman stars in the 1967 film version of the 1963 novel *The Graduate* by Charles Webb. Pure American collegiate style, the beaming Los Angeles sun gives a dreamy feel to Benjamin's conservative wardrobe. The movie portrays a young man seduced by an older woman (Anne Bancroft) – his naivety represented at the beginning by his uptight Ivy League style, but his rite-of-passage affair with Mrs Robinson transforms his look into one more of ease and confidence. A cooler Braddock emerges in T-shirts, gym shoes and parka – this East-meets-West Coast style is perennially referenced by designers. Could there be a better accessory than Mrs Robinson?

Lester Diamond from Casino

Martin Scorsese's 1995 gangster flick *Casino* is a full-on feast of 1970s and 1980s bling, set in Las Vegas. Lester Diamond is the spivvy pimp who steals the limelight from the larger characters with his O.T.T. lounge lizard attire. Diamond is pure 1970s Gucci jet set; leeching money off Sharon Stone's character Ginger, he fritters it away on drugs, fast cars and his wardrobe.

His best scene is in a restaurant where he is wearing a flared white jean suit with Gucci red and green epaulettes and matching cuffs. Diamond is total con-man cool – all suede tasselled loafers. Even though he wasn't the slickest or most groomed character in the film, he makes it onto the list because he leaves you wanting more and waiting to see what he's going to wear next.

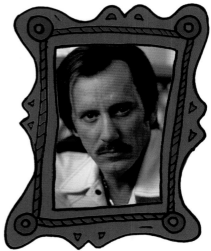

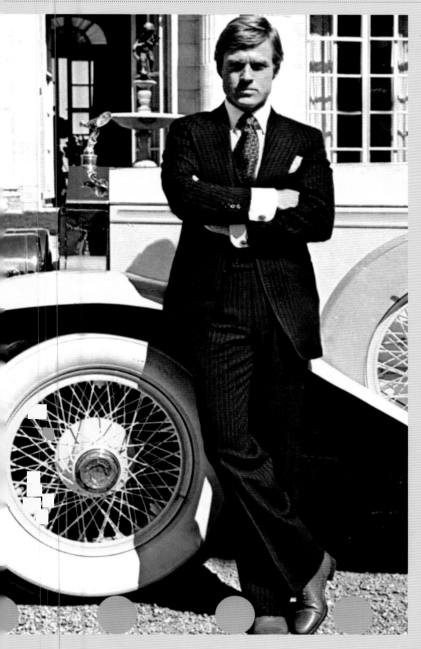

Jay Gatsby from The Great Gatsby

You have to admire a man whose wardrobe can stir this kind of emotion: "It makes me sad because I've never seen such, such beautiful shirts before," says Daisy, the object of Jay Gatsby's affection. F Scott Fitzgerald's 1925 novel *The Great Gatsby* epitomizes the great Jazz Age and everything stylish and sophisticated about the era. In the story, Jay Gatsby aims to win the heart of past love, Daisy Buchanan, by acquiring wealth and style.

The most famous film adaptation was Jack Clayton's 1974 version starring Robert Redford as Jay Gatsby with a wardrobe by Ralph Lauren. All the clothes came from his Polo line, with the exception of the pink suit specially designed for the film and an old-fashioned striped wool bathing costume. Even though the film has a dash of the 1970s about it, Jay's style never dates.

Gordon Gekko from Wall Street

Michael Douglas as Gordon Gekko, the main character from the 1987 film *Wall Street*, is the only man who can truly carry off the yuppie uniform of contrast-collar shirt and wide, striped braces (suspenders). Sleeves rolled up and pleated trousers is a smart look made real by a man who ruthlessly pursued money.

Costume designer Ellen Mirojnick designed Gekko's look, choosing Alan Flusser to tailor the suits and Alex Kabbaz to custom-make the shirts. These were based on a shirt Kabbaz had designed for Tom Wolfe in the early 1980s. Flusser saw the shirt and asked Tom if he would mind if he used the idea for Michael Douglas's movie wardrobe. The blue shirt with the white contrast collar and French cuff became known as the "Gekko Shirt". Slicked-back hair and a ridiculous level of self-confidence and arrogance makes Gekko the anti-hero of the 1980s. Greed looks good!

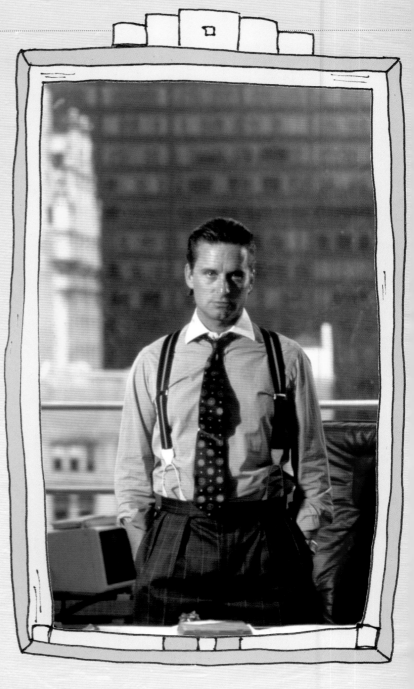

Dickie Greenleaf and Tom Ripley from The Talented Mr Ripley

Director Anthony Minghella turned the 1955 psychological thriller by Patricia Highsmith into a film in 1999, starring Jude Law as the rich and confident Dickie Greenleaf and Matt Damon as wannabe Tom Ripley. Focusing on young, wealthy, spoilt Americans escaping the constraints of family expectations, *The Talented Mr Ripley* is a very sunny and blonde film of perfect summer dressing. Both lead characters have been included as they virtually morph into one when Tom starts to borrow Dickie's clothes and eventually takes over his entire persona.

Tom starts out as an awkward and aspiring young man wearing thick corduroy in the Italian sun, but gradually moulds himself on Dickie's image by mixing old-world American clothes and items he has picked up in Italy. The Chic Geek loves the duffle coats at the end of the movie. According to costume designer Ann Roth, "If you were one of the glamour people you were allowed to run away from school and you ended up in Paris or on the Riviera. And that's what *The Talented Mr Ripley* is about. Dickie's wealth is casually expressed and, since he's avoiding his family, perhaps tattered a bit around the edges; his Gucci loafers may be worn through, and his tailor-made outfits may be ratty. But he still looks classy and stylish. Ripley is another matter... He comes from Princeton, and he's very American East Coast, but from Sears." *The Talented Mr Ripley* has become a modern style classic, mixing vintage 1950s glamour in a timeless and contemporary way. Favourite line of the film has to be: "I always thought it'd be better to be a fake somebody than a real nobody."

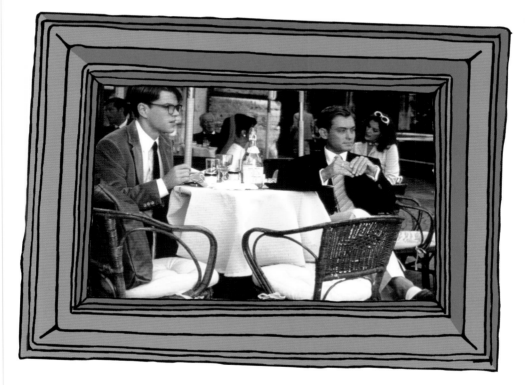

Sherlock Holmes

Sherlock Holmes epitomizes quirky Victoriana. The deerstalker hat, cape and pipe provide us with the defining dramatic image of the Victorian male. Sir Arthur Conan Doyle's fictional detective solidly represents the foggy drama of nineteenth-century London. A man of intelligence and independent financial means, Holmes is defiantly uppercrust and flaunts this in his attire. In the novels, he usually wears a fedora or a bowler hat, and not the deerstalker. He is described as having a "cat-like love of personal cleanliness" and normally dresses in conventional tweeds and a frock coat, wearing a dressing gown in the privacy of Baker Street. A towering and authoritative figure, you wouldn't want to mess with this stick-wielding martial arts expert.

Captain Von Trapp from The Sound of Music

It is the smart and dapper Tyrolean flavour that most appeals about Captain Von Trapp. Christopher Plummer played the role of the Captain in the 1965 film *The Sound of Music* opposite Julie Andrews. His strict, disciplinarian military style is evident in his grey and forest-green suits and smart leather boots. This traditional Germanic style is surprisingly contemporary with three or four buttoned felt or tweed jackets, topped with a feathered mountaineer hat. Luckily he never let Maria run anything up on her sewing machine, otherwise he may not have made it onto our list.

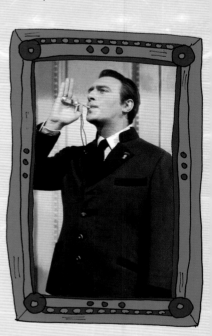

Bertie Wooster

Written by PG Wodehouse, Bertie Wooster is the narrator of 10 novels and over 30 short stories. An English gentleman who leaves common sense to the commoners, Bertie is a member of the "idle rich" and spends his time taking supper at his members club, Drones, or getting into feeble-minded scrapes. He displays the full gamut of a gentleman's dress during the 1930s. When Bertie catches his valet Meadowes stealing his silk socks, he sacks him and sends for another from the agency. Jeeves arrives and can be thanked for putting Bertie onto The Chic Geek's list. Jeeves is the knowledge behind the pompous dressing etiquette of English society, taking all the effort away from Bertie. From plus fours to white tie, the new valet makes sure Bertie looks his best at all times.

Jeeves: *"Pardon me for asking, sir, but are you proposing to appear in public in those garments?"*

Bertie: *"Well, certainly Jeeves. What – a bit vivid, do you think?"*

Jeeves: *"Not necessarily sir. I am told that M. Freddie 'He's a Riot' Flowerdew often appears on the music-hall stage in comparable attire."*

THE ULTIMATE CHIC GEEKS

Jarvis Cocker

His lanky frame, dirty thick-framed spectacles and greasy hair turned Jarvis Cocker into a style icon for the 1990s. Lead singer of the British band Pulp, he fronted one of the coolest and artiest indie groups of the decade, his tall, weedy, stick-insect-like body personifying the awkward and difficult boy who stood out. His lyrics documented his time at art school and consisted of honest social observations. Twirling his hand and pointing, he was shielded from the bullies in his skinny corduroy suits, which looked like lucky charity-shop finds.

Cocker turned the school teacher/librarian/elbow-patches look cool, but with an element of knowing. In 2002 he said, "It's all gone a bit weird with clothes now, hasn't it? When you used to find a jacket or whatever in Oxfam, part of the thing was wondering who wore it before you, what the history was. It's all gone, that. Now, everyone's paying a fortune for jeans that look like a tramp slept in them for four weeks." This indie geek is a great example of vintage style, mixing things up and working what you have shape-wise. He puts great thought into his clothes, but has stayed true to his instantly recognizable style. Jarvis Cocker is truly in a "different class".

Live Aid
David Bowie

David Bowie is so huge in terms of image that you have to break him down. He's had so many different personas over the years it could be hard to choose one that stands out, but when it come to male style that translates, The Chic Geek had to pick the early 1980s. This was smooth Bowie, handsome Bowie and suave Bowie. Hair dyed blond, colour on his skin, it was the healthiest and chicest he ever looked.

The rockabilly quiff, the nod to the Zoot era, Bowie used the suit to launch a new, pop-sounding chapter in his music career. He put on his red shoes and sang the blues on the *Let's Dance* album and wore suits that were a completely new shape: short double-breasted jackets with very pronounced shoulders and a slanted top pocket and wide trousers.

In the "China Girl" video he wears a tiny, four-button, pastel double-breasted jacket with a shirt and tie, his tousled blond hair bouncing on his head. He continued the theme throughout his *Serious Moonlight* tour, but the 1985 performance of "Heroes" at Wembley Stadium in London for Live Aid is his strongest image from this time. Swaying in an ice-blue suit, with white buttons, patterned lemon tie and white shirt, he appears timeless. He even pulls off white socks, and the jacket's shoulders are so strong they turn the top half of his body into an almost-perfect square. Bowie has never looked better.

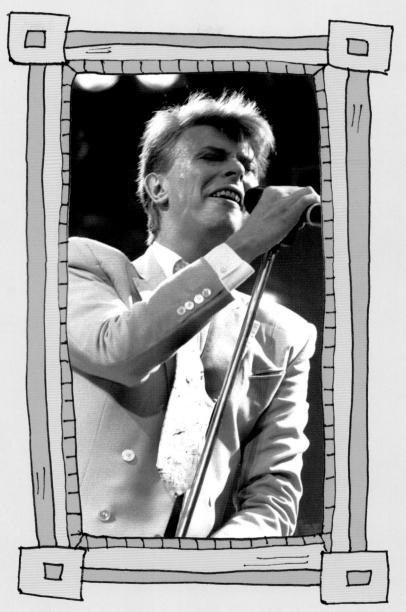

Bryan Ferry

After a brief flirtation with 1970s glam, Ferry settled into a lifetime of smart suits. Lead singer of British band Roxy Music, he started the Robert Palmer thing of rock stars wearing suits and slim ties on stage. Collaborating with tailor Antony Price, his long thin frame was, and still is, perfect for wearing a suit. His late 1970s suits had a spivvy quality and were Zoot-inspired, especially when paired with Ferry's skinny moustache in the "Let's Stick Together" video.

Antony Price didn't just tailor Ferry's suits, he also collaborated with Roxy Music on stage sets, costumes and album covers, creating a strong look that defined the 1980s. Draped in Jerry Hall (until she was stolen by Mick Jagger), Ferry carried off Price's acid suiting, tightly waisted and square-shouldered. "Secretly, I wanted to look like Jimi Hendrix, but I could never quite pull it off," he once said. In later years Ferry has managed to mix town and country, pulling out the old black suit and skinny tie to perform in, while becoming something of a classic and tasteful English gent off-stage. Ferry is a great example of a man who has aged well.

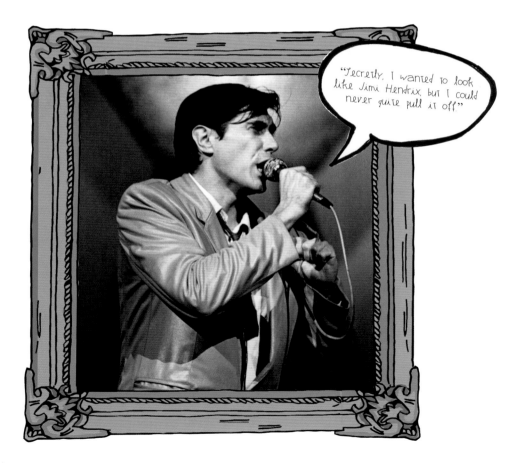

"Secretly, I wanted to look like Jimi Hendrix, but I could never quite pull it off."

Jude Law

British actor Jude Law is the modern poster boy of a stylish movie star. He can wear anything from a tracksuit to a dinner suit and has the swagger and good-looking arrogance to carry it off. He's been the face of campaigns for Dunhill and Dior fragrance and is a perfect example of the man wearing the clothes and not the clothes wearing the man.

But good looks are just one of his attributes. He's not perfect or overly groomed, with a thinning hairline and slightly dishevelled bed-hair, but he's got the cheeky roguishness, confidence and ease that come with being stylish. It's the shots of him at home in Primrose Hill, London, just popping out for a pint of milk, that show his real style: jeans, trainers (sneakers), man-cleavage T-shirt just thrown on, but still looking cool.

Jude Law doesn't make massive style statements, but he always sits on the right side of trendy cool. It helps that he is very handsome and has a great body, but there are plenty of movie stars with the same credentials and none of the flair. On screen he even managed to carry off a moustache as Dr Watson in *Sherlock Holmes* and his role as Dickie Greenleaf in *The Talented Mr Ripley* is still resurrected every summer as a look to emulate. But as he says, "Face it, I didn't become famous until I took my clothes off."

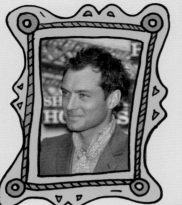

Pharrell Williams

The American recording artist, producer, musician and fashion designer Pharrell Williams is the perfect chic geek, even calling his group N.E.R.D. He knows what it's like to be different and frankly, he doesn't care. From his customized Hermès bags to his own fashion label, Pharrell likes trying new things and mixing it up a bit. A sartorial sponge, he takes references from everywhere, recently describing a cape in one of his collections as "Purdey mixed with a bit of Malcolm McLaren".

Pharrell is co-founder of fashion labels Billionaire Boys Club and Ice Cream, alongside Japanese designer Nigo of A Bathing Ape; he has also designed glasses and jewellery for Louis Vuitton. His style could be described as street, but he is also very eclectic and the more you study him the more you notice his classic, dressier pieces. At school he was the cool geek, the guy who had enough confidence to go with his gut; as he says, "Fashion has to reflect who you are, what you feel at the moment, and where you're going. It doesn't have to be bright, doesn't have to be loud. Just has to be *you*." Pharrell is a great example of playful confidence and he wears his well.

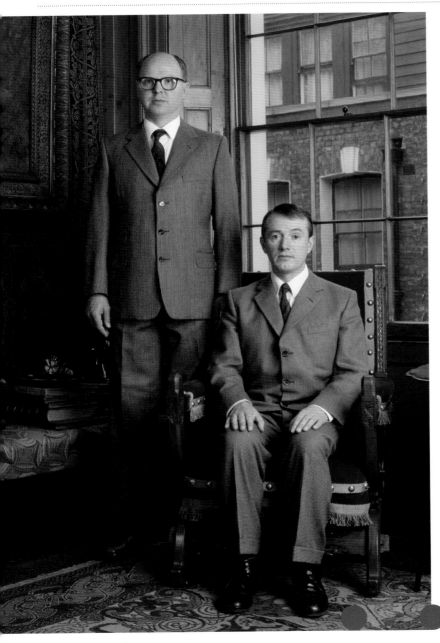

Gilbert & George

Two for the price of one, contemporary artists Gilbert & George always come as a pair. They met at Central Saint Martins College of Art and Design in London in the 1960s and have been inseparable ever since. Gilbert (the small one) is Italian-born while George (the tall one) is English. They are based in London's trendy Spitalfields, where they get most of the inspiration for their work, including giant stained-glass style montages of human excrement and other bodily fluids. "Nothing happens in the world that doesn't happen in the East End," they say.

Unlike many other artists, you never see them in the "process" of making art, and they are always immaculately turned out in identical tweed suits. Most of their suits are made by David London of Hackney Road, who once dressed some of the nattiest gents in East London's Bethnal Green and has since retired.

Gilbert & George use themselves and their image as a kind of "living sculpture" – it would be interesting to know how much of their lives are real and how much is an act. The two artists can be quite disconcerting, but have a dry sense of humour that is reflected in their hugely successful artworks. They hate what they call the "uniform" of jeans: "We are more offended by blue jeans than anything else. They are appalling. It's a uniform," says Gilbert. "It's the fear of standing out," agrees George, "The fear of being different."

David Hockney

Artist David Hockney is great at catching the zeitgeist. Just look at his painting *Mr and Mrs Clark and Percy*; it's a perfect snapshot of 1970s glamour – the shag pile, the chair and the clothes. Only a truly stylish person would pick up on those details, and with such skill.

Born under the grey skies of Bradford and moving to the bright light of California, Hockney is not only a painter, but also a photographer, draftsman and he has even turned his hand to the iPad. A master of colour and line, designers such as Christopher Bailey at Burberry and Paul Smith have referenced his style in their collections.

Hockney is famous for wearing different-coloured socks and thickly rimmed Le Corbusier-style circular glasses; he has always cultivated a striking look. From his student days at the Royal College of Art in London to poolside in LA, Hockney knew the power of image in art. His bright blond mop of hair, black glasses and large windowpane-check suits create an image that has stood the test of time.

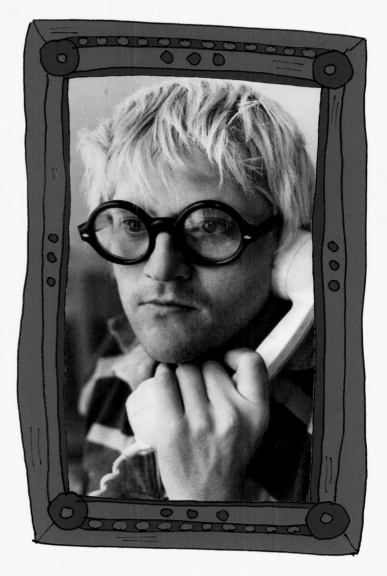

Mick Jagger

The Rolling Stone is in a category of his own. He can look ridiculous (think spandex leggings and sweatshirts), but because he's Mick Jagger he gets away with it – he's the only man who can work a unitard (just!). Bouncing around on stage like a hyperactive toddler, Jagger is a ball of energy whose style has been influencing men's fashion for decades. "Very early on we did the same thing young bands are now doing," he explained in an interview. "We wore clothes very similar to what we wore offstage because we didn't have any money and that was the look. It wasn't until the end of the 1960s, when the Rolling Stones were playing 50,000-seat arenas, that the band began to wear more 'eye-catching' stuff."

A man of wealth and taste, Jagger became a client of the influential British fashion designer Ossie Clark in the late 1960s. Clark made some of Jagger's stage costumes, such as a python-skin jumpsuit that was designed to unzip onstage for the Rolling Stones' 1973 tour. A famous image of Jagger is one taken on his wedding day in a white Yves Saint Laurent suit marrying his first wife Bianca.

With Jagger, though, it's more than the clothes; it's the lips, the hair and the vacant look. Running on the adrenaline of sex, drugs and rock 'n' roll, he is a chameleon, with the only thing to stay constant being his sinewy frame.

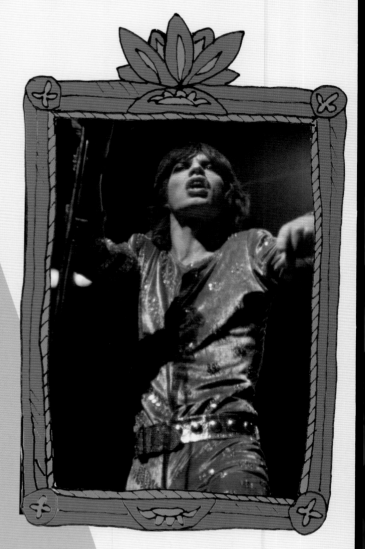

Early Elton John

This is Elton John pre-Gianni Versace; Elton John before he wore black jackets embellished with Swarovski Medusas. This is Elton when he was balding, 1970s Elton, the Elton of quilted satin and giant *Tommy*-style platform boots. The man looked amazing: rhinestone jumpsuits, matching coloured bowler hats, Donald Duck outfits... it was so silly, and it was so cool. This was true superstar showmanship.

Elton was outrageous, but his outfits were so beautifully designed and made that, looking back, the images of him just keep getting better. He is a stylish example of the excesses of the decade. According to John Reid (Elton's ex-manager), "I encouraged his outrageousness at first. He was 23 and very unworldly when we first met... over the next four years his clothes got brighter, his glasses got bigger... each show he wanted more and more."

For the honour of being the 1,662nd entertainer to have a gold star on Hollywood Boulevard's Walk of Fame, Elton had a pair of star-shaped specs specially made to go with his bespoke outfit which boasted over 50 stars, complete with names. Around this time his shopaholic nature and low boredom threshold was becoming apparent. In a quote from 1973 he said, "I always have a pair of glasses to go with every outfit I own. At the moment I have 50 pairs, which I carry around with me... and guard them with my life!... I've had this red streak in my hair for four months now, which is a long time for me, so I'll soon get it changed to another colour. My boots are far less outrageous than they used to be because I went off them... I get my suits made for me – I would buy shop clothes, but they'd wear out too quickly because I'm really heavy on clothes. I love jewellery too...." The Lady Gaga of his day, each outfit was as outlandish as the next. The songs weren't bad either.

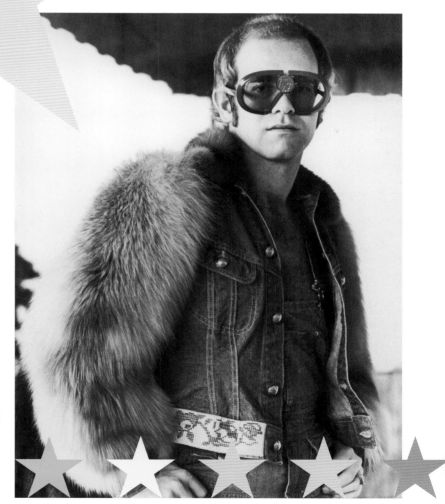

Paul Newman

Oscar-winning legend Paul Newman had an incredibly good-looking innocence. His mother said in a 1959 interview, "In a way, it was a shame to waste so much beauty on a boy," but this boy also knew how to dress.

The original American boy-next-door, Newman didn't have a signature style but made everything look simple and easy. It was so simple you didn't really notice it, and that's a true gift. He had an old-fashioned refinement; a working-class humility that endeared him to many. A man who never forgot where he came from, he was natural and didn't need the frivolities of fashion to stand out.

He was of his era but also timeless, and none of his images have dated; simple combinations of white shirts and slim ties, and off-duty looks of American classics, such as cowboy shirts and jeans, focused on the man himself and the characters he portrayed. Even playing gritty characters such as Lucas Jackson from *Cool Hand Luke* couldn't dull those trademark blue eyes. He never seemed to be aware of his own beauty or image, or if he did, then he really was a great actor. He once said, "I was always a character actor. I just looked like Little Red Riding Hood."

Newman was a philanthropist long before it was all about gaining exposure for your career. He started his food business in 1982 and it has generated more than $300 million for charities. What's more, he never stood on ceremony: he was his own man. On his 75th birthday he burnt his tuxedo because he "was done with formality". Newman may have had the looks, but it takes true style to carry off a bottle of salad dressing.

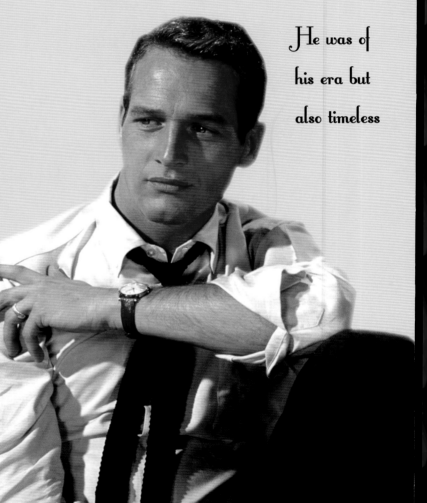

He was of his era but also timeless

HRH The Prince of Wales

The true test of a stylish gentleman is to ask yourself if you've even seen him looking bad – the answer for Prince Charles would have to be "no". But while he's not the most excitingly dressed character, the devil is in the detail. Considering the number of times he has been seen and photographed over the years, it is testimony to his own sense of style that he is hard to fault. Like his mother, the Prince is above fashion and trends. He always dresses correctly for the occasion, but with his own touches – the small knot on the tie and the signet ring – and continues the tradition of royal men not only dressing well, but also enjoying it.

Prince Charles is famous for his Savile Row suits. Mr Hitchcock, head tailor at Anderson & Sheppard, confirms that His Royal Highness has his own exclusive cloth, Balmoral Tweed, and that they cut to his own personal taste. This is usually double-breasted with a peaked lapel, natural curves and fewer seams, which Anderson & Sheppard have perfected over the last 30 years.

Prince Charles flies the flag for British design and quality and is a walking advertisement for investment shopping, wearing the same clothes for decades. He is frequently seen in a winter coat, modelled on one owned by his great-uncle the Duke of Windsor, which he has had for over 20 years. His shirts and ties are from Turnbull & Asser and he has his dressing room laid out like a tailor's shop. Keeping up with the current trend for recycling, cufflinks have been made out of parts from the engine of the Prince's former Aston Martin. He said, "I even have a pair of shoes made from bales of leather salvaged from an eighteenth-century wreck off the southwest of Britain. They are totally indestructible and will see me out."

You could argue that Prince Charles's privileged upbringing accounts for his style, but his exquisite taste extends beyond wealth – you only have to look at his home and garden at Highgrove to see that. He dresses like a true British monarch, carrying on the traditions and indulgences of his forebears.

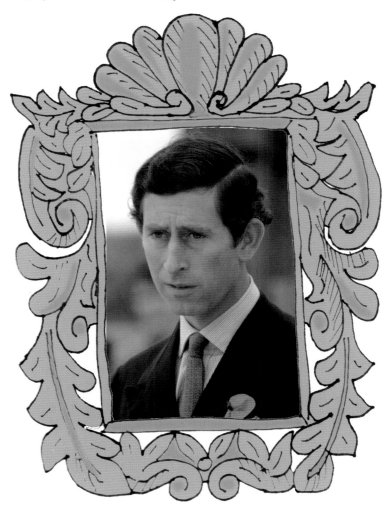

Andy Warhol

American Pop artist Andy Warhol knew cool when he saw it, then bottled it and made a fortune selling it. He also knew how to use his image as a magical tool in a new era of celebrity, which he pioneered. Obsessed with his appearance, the trademark white wig and sunglasses made him instantly recognizable, but he never allowed anyone through that veneer. He once said, "I'd prefer to remain a mystery. I never like to give my background and, anyway, I make it all up different every time I'm asked. It's not just that it's part of my image not to tell everything, it's just that I forget what I said the day before, and I have to make it all up over again."

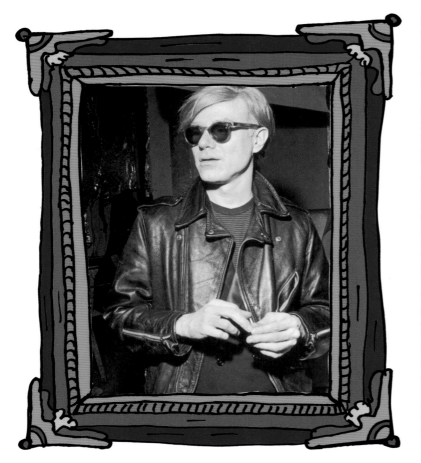

Warhol thought himself ugly due to a skin condition, and so he had cabinets full of beauty products. He thought that if he surrounded himself with beauty, he too would become beautiful. A total voyeur, he would go out nearly every night to observe. "Fashion… wasn't what you wore someplace anymore. It was the whole reason for going," he said.

He started out as a fashion illustrator in New York, sketching shoes for women's magazines and department store advertising, and was one of the first artists to embrace commercialism. His "Factory" studio became the epicentre of alternative 1960s New York, where he developed his Beatnik uniform of skinny black jeans, stripy turtlenecks and a black leather jacket; oh, and of course, the sunglasses. He famously once said, "Think rich, look poor." A complete enigma, nobody seemed to know the real Warhol, but we can take a lot from him in terms of his simple but strict style. In the late 1970s and 1980s he moved to a more preppy jackets-and-ties image. He religiously wore "Creation" style shoes from Italian brand Salvatore Ferragamo.

It took Sotheby's ten days to auction the 10,000 items left in Warhol's house after his death, most of it random stuff he'd picked up at flea markets. The auction grossed more than US$20 million. Warhol took style to the grave: lying in his coffin, he was dressed in a black cashmere suit, a paisley tie, a platinum wig and sunglasses. What a way to go! He once said, "I never think that people die. They just go to department stores."

Tom Wolfe

American author and journalist Tom Wolfe is an uptight vision in white. It takes commitment, not to mention dry-cleaning bills, to be able to wear his famous white suit, day in and day out. The story goes that Wolfe bought his first white suit planning to wear it in the summer in the style of a Southern gentlemen. However, he found the suit too hot for the summer, so he began to wear it in the winter instead. This caused quite a sensation, so he adopted the white suit as his trademark in 1962.

His own personal uniform (a devil to cut because, according to his Italian tailor, you can scarcely see the chalk marks), he sometimes wears the suits with a waistcoat as a three-piece, with a matching white tie, white homburg hat and two-tone shoes. A social voyeur, Wolfe has said that the white suit disarms the people he observes, making him in their eyes, "a man from Mars, the man who didn't know anything and was eager to know." When it comes to his appearance, Wolfe usually quotes Mark Twain: "The last thing in the world I want to be is conspicuous, but I do want to be noticed."

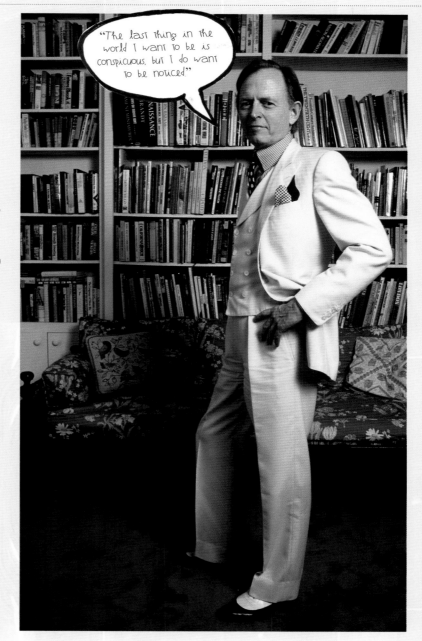

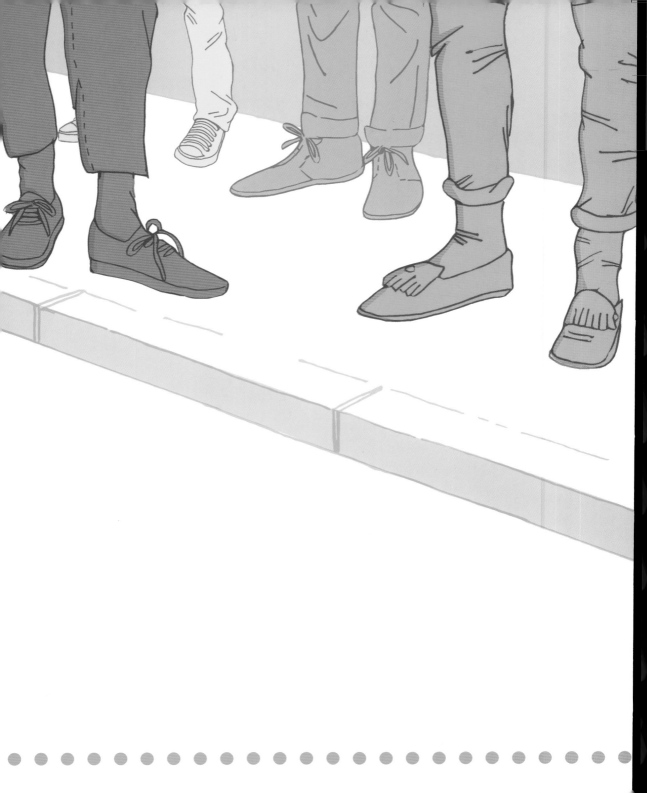

2

StreetGeek

Take a guy straight off the catwalk or from the pages of a glossy magazine, put him on the street and he would look completely over-styled; it just doesn't work. Reality has a different level of fashion, so when it comes to everyday life, things have to be slightly diluted for them to look convincing in the "real" world. Welcome to the StreetGeek, The Chic Geek's roving eye, where he takes snapshots of the coolest guys on the streets of the world's chicest cities.

This chapter shows examples of stylish-looking, real men, photographed on the street going about their daily lives, and then dissects what is great about their looks. Lots of men will see another guy and know instinctively that he looks good but aren't sure exactly what it is about them that works. The Chic Geek analyzes each guy in detail in order to illuminate how their styles can be copied or integrated into your own look.

It is interesting to see how many varied looks there are and how different parts of one city have a completely different look from another. Our supposedly globalized world still has subtle style and fashion nuances. Things like the weather and cultural ideas introduce a new take on contemporary male style and inspiration can be gained from all these exotic locations.

Over the next few pages you will see everyday sartorial excellence in London, Paris, Milan, Stockholm and Tokyo. So, get out there guys and get papped by the The Chic Geek!

LONDON

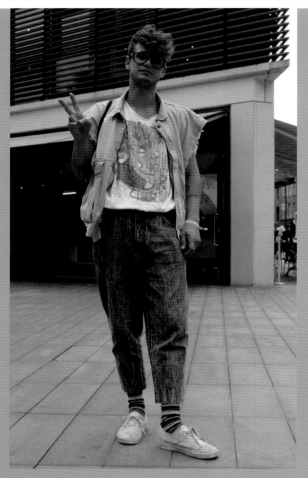

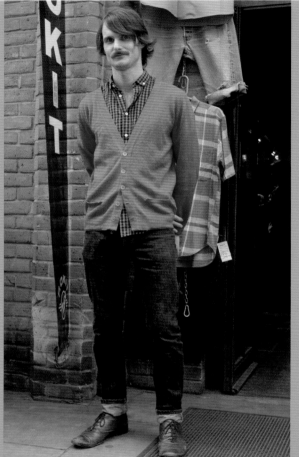

▲ This is pure East London, too cool for school. The acid-wash vintage jeans have a generous shape which gives a new silhouette, away from the predictable skinny. The cut-off jacket by Rokit goes with the 1980s jean. Large-frame glasses by Cesare Paciotti and a high-top trainer (sneaker) on the T-shirt continue the 1980s look. I like the pumps and stripy socks. This is cool fun.

▲ I just love this colour. The bright primary red works with everything; black, white and this petrol-blue gingham Colin has teamed it with. This strong red works well in a cardigan as you can play with the level of colour; it would be too blocky in a sweater or jumper. Colin has undone the bottom two buttons to show how you can alter the intensity of the colour by breaking it up differently. The jeans are nicely tapered but not too tight, with a large but perfectly proportioned turn-up (cuff) matched with the slightly bashed-up, brown shoes.

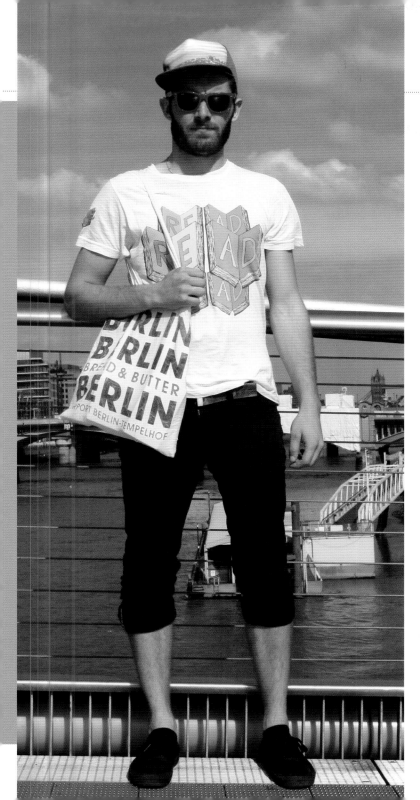

◄ This is trendy with a capital "T". Sacha has played with bold colour with the hat, the sunglasses and the Marc Jacobs T-shirt, yet it works and he doesn't look like a fashion victim. The most interesting thing is the American Apparel trousers, skinny and cut off below the knee like capri pants, but they still look masculine – the beard probably helps! A new trouser shape: take note. The bag is from Bread & Butter in Berlin.

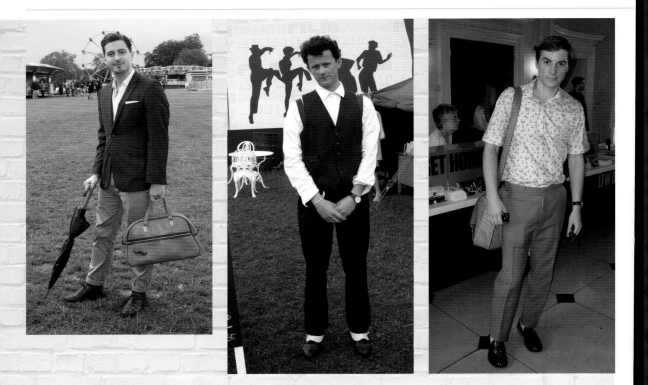

▲ David's jacket is great with the smart *Mad Men*-style pocket square, but it's the Bryl-creemed hair that really makes it vintage. Nice turn-ups (cuffs) on the camel trousers. A bowling-bag style leather bag and blue umbrella make the finishing gentlemanly touch.

▲ This is vintage shabby chic. Ivo is wearing evening clothes but, by not wearing a necktie or bow-tie, it works for daytime. The spats are a nice detail on the shoes and complement the white shirt. His trousers have a tuxedo stripe down the side and pleats at the front.

▲ Barnaby here has a very individual retro look going on. He looks like somebody's dad on holiday, circa 1970s. The printed shirt is actually new, by Dunhill, but looks vintage in that washed way. Short-sleeve shirts always have a retro quality. The trousers, by Lou Dalton, are that putty colour much beloved in the 1970s and are just the right length to flatter the highly polished, reddish, antiqued loafers.

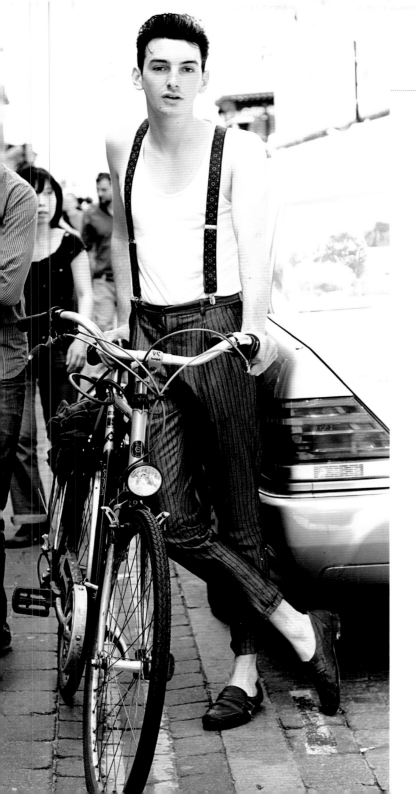

◄ Such a good look. Where to start? The high-waisted pleated tapered trousers that look almost shiny or wet; the stretched skinny vest matched with patterned regular-sized braces (suspenders); the slip-on shoes all accessorized with the bike? This is one of those looks where you are not sure if a lot of thought went into it or not, which is what makes it so cool.

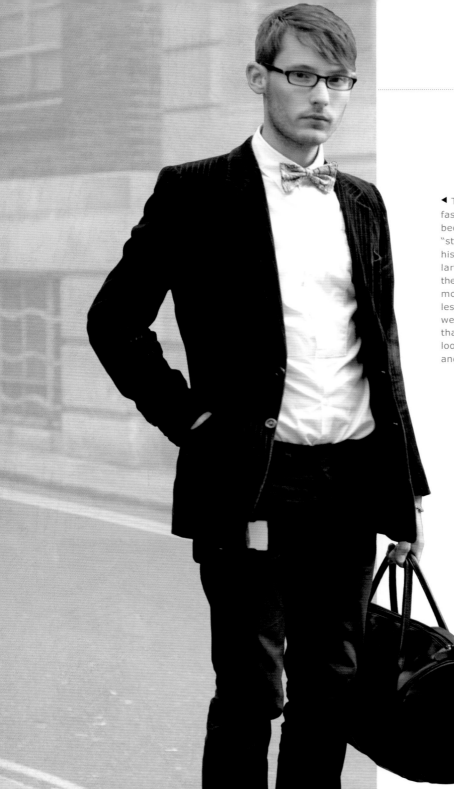

◄ The bow-tie is now a ubiquitous fashion statement and as such has become a little too common in the "style" arena. Here, John has teamed his bow-tie with a dress shirt and a large-wale corduroy jacket. Adding the corduroy allows the look to be more daytime and professor-like, less evening dress. I like the way he wears his ID on his trousers rather than his lapel, so as not to ruin the look. The small holdall is a nice size and shape.

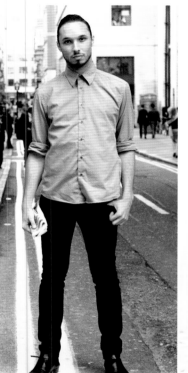

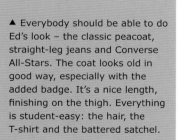

▲ Leaving your shirt untucked used to be only for lager louts, but because Paul's shirt finishes short and it is fitted and buttoned-up, he gets away with it. The colour of the shirt and black fitted trousers also perfectly reflect his skin and hair colour.

▲ It is harder to pull off an evening jacket during the day if it is in a dark colour as it can make you look overdressed. Harry's is a nice cream tone – it's only the shawl collar and single black button that tells you it's eveningwear. Combined with the tousled hair and bracelets, this is a relaxed way to do a day-to-evening look.

▲ Everybody should be able to do Ed's look – the classic peacoat, straight-leg jeans and Converse All-Stars. The coat looks old in good way, especially with the added badge. It's a nice length, finishing on the thigh. Everything is student-easy: the hair, the T-shirt and the battered satchel.

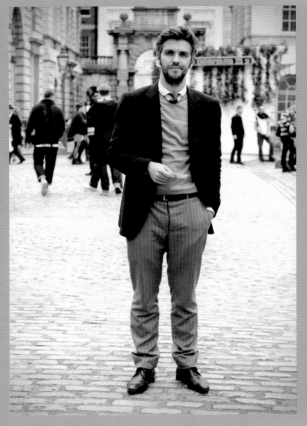

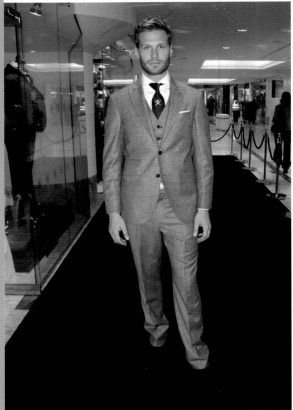

▲ Men's Fashion Day at London Fashion Week is a perfect example of the difference between fashion and style. While there is always a lot of fashion milling around, it is the stylish people who stand out. Andrew here has kept it tight. I like the way he has layered a T-shirt over the shirt instead of a jumper and then pulled the tie forward thus slightly lowering the T-shirt. The taupe colour of the shirt complements not only the pin-striped trousers but also the colour of his hair and beard. He looks handsomely stylish.

▲ You don't get many guys looking like this in Canary Wharf. Okay, this is a bit of a cheat. Freddy is a model wearing Hackett for a shop opening but we had to take the picture. Jeremy Hackett is so good at this soft, woolly, just-the-right-thickness tweed suit. This three-piece is a perfect suit shape.

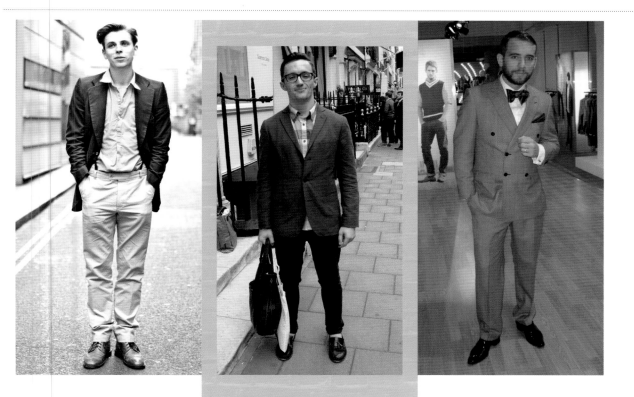

▲ Dandyism at its finest. Henry has that slightly nonchalant air of creased formality that only an Englishman can carry off. The rolled-shoulder, billiard-green velvet jacket has been contrasted with claret-coloured braces (suspenders). He has made what would be a traditional outfit of beige chinos, light blue shirt and brown brogues stand out in a seemingly effortless way.

▲ Jaime has chosen a nice palette of greens and blues and the checked shirt is Uniqlo. He has something of the Clark Kent vibe about him in a good way, with his tightly parted hair and glasses, but he's managed to yoof it up a bit with fitted black jeans and tasselled loafers sans socks. The jacket fits perfectly and he's only used the middle button – classy. He looks relaxed but fashionably attired.

▲ This is old-school dapper. While the general idea is to dress down these days, there is a small contingent of men doing the opposite and going über-dressed. Graeme here is wearing a vintage-inspired, double-breasted Prince of Wales check suit with the full kit and caboodle of bow-tie, pocket square, cufflinks and polished shoes. If this picture was in black and white, you'd be hard pushed to guess the year. Timeless.

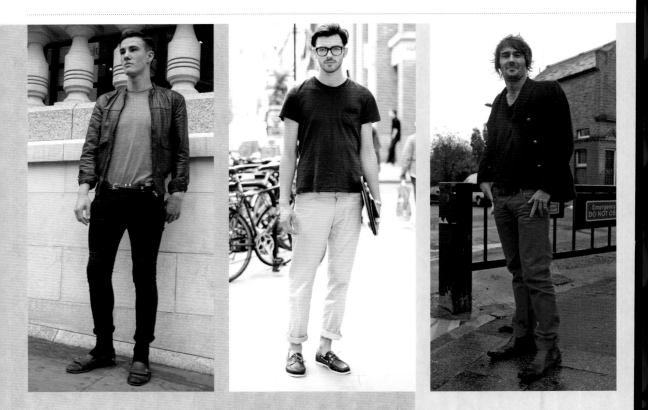

▲ This is one of the best street geeks we've seen. Ross has really got it going on here. The hair is immaculate, Bryl-creemed to perfection, but it's the touches that make it: the rolled sleeves on the jacket and the T-shirt tucked into the jeans, which makes the belt visible, looks smarter and shows off a flat stomach (if you have it)! The retro shoes are from Beyond Retro and rolling up the jeans works so well with the socks. Sublime.

▲ This is pure chic geek: the glasses, the rolled-up trousers, even the posture. Check out the oversized glasses and boat shoes; this is a really nice summer look for the city. Simple, not too much going on. It works.

▲ This is quite a traditional look. The double-breasted jacket and bright red trousers are very English gentleman, but Julian gives it a rougher edge with the hair and V-neck T-shirt. Fashion has returned to English classics like the bright trousers. The belt and shoes are by Paul Smith.

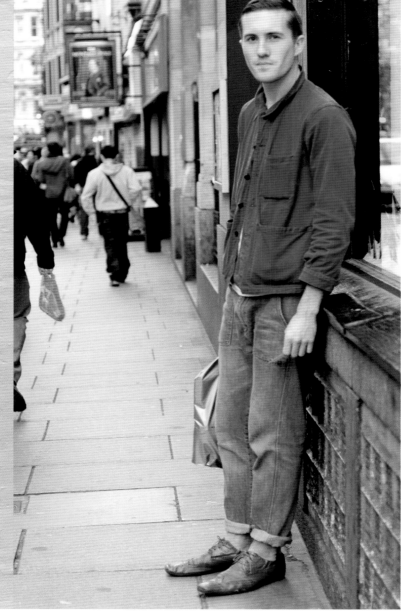

▶ This is a great jacket, very Chairman Mao. The colour is inky-strong and the proportions are good; look at the baggy pockets and the way it is really short on Joleyn's arms. It's all very "Comrades Unite" worker chic. The short arms are echoed by the turn-ups (cuffs) on the jeans and great reddish brown lace-ups. The neat hair keeps the look from being too artistic.

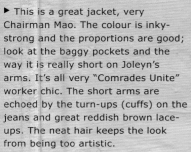

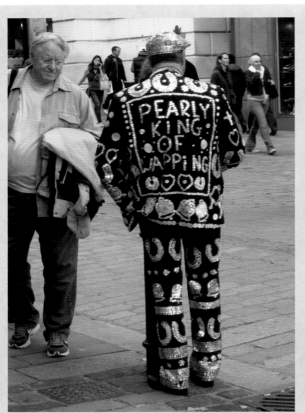

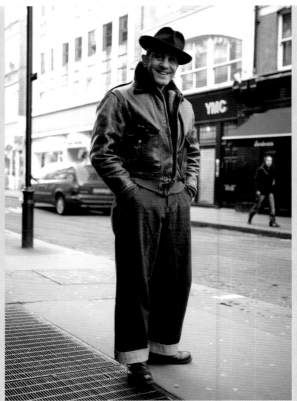

▲ If you want real London street style, look no further than this guy! This classic cockney "Pearly King of Wapping" was busy selling poppies to raise money for the Poppy Appeal. I just love this outfit – the mother-of-pearl buttons sewn into designs of bells, hearts and horseshoes – it's London's own traditional costume. He continues the tradition of Pearly Kings and Queens by raising money for charity and this style of sewing on buttons has influenced many designers, particularly Alexander McQueen. Always reminds me of Mary Poppins.

▲ Christos looks like a character from an American comic, very Dick Tracy. It gives a 1940s feeling: the shearling flight jacket, wide Zoot-suit-style trousers with large turn-ups (cuffs) and polished army boots, all finished with a great hat. The look is really fun – you're just waiting for him to start jiving!

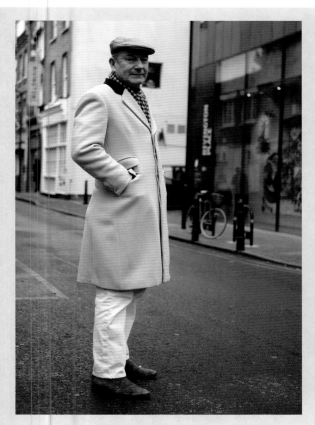

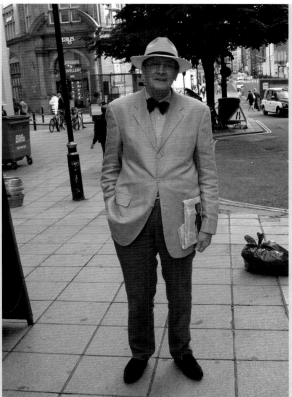

▲ This is what we label "Trotter chic", the classic "gin and jag" look pioneered in the 1980s. Eddie is pure working-class smart: the gingham scarf, a small flash of Prince of Wales check suit, the tweed flat cap. The pastel lemon Crombie with claret collar is a timeless dandy piece. An amazing array of textures, colours and patterns, and it works because it has a sense of humour. This goes into the Hall of Fame of Englishmen's looks.

▲ Charles here is beyond fashion. This is the classic summer look of the English gentleman: Panama hat, linen jacket, dickie bow and suede loafers. Charles said he had had the clothes for a long time, which is testament to the ethos of the traditional Englishman's look – buy well and it'll last a lifetime.

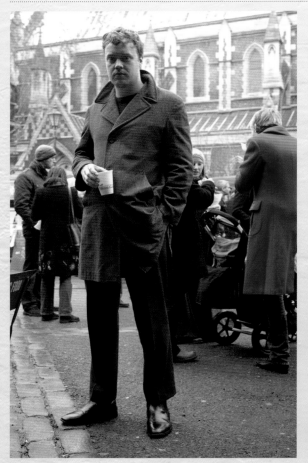

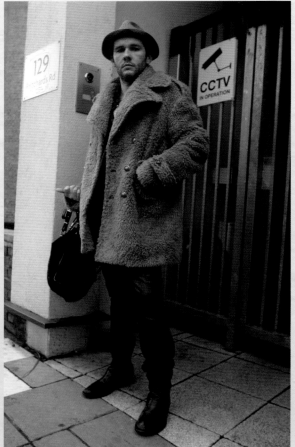

▲ You'll never find this look anywhere but Britain. John is one part Teddy Boy, one part Michael Caine. This is shabby chic, scruffy almost, yet he has a finesse, an attitude, that speaks cool. The look is timeless: a nice navy round-neck waffle sweater, a single-breasted coat in a grey check with the collar edged up and brown slacks. He could have been out all night and you can imagine a whole story around him. If he quiffed his hair slightly you would think this was taken in the 1950s, yet the look remains contemporary and not a vintage pastiche. What's it all about, Alfie?

▲ I like how Bryan here is wearing some heavy-hitting designer names such as Burberry Prorsum, Fendi and Dior Homme yet has made a street look of it. The coat is the choicest piece from the autumn-winter 2010 Burberry Prorsum collection – the kind of coat you'd dream about finding in a vintage shop. This is thrown-on luxe dressing, very rock-star chic! The bag by Fendi, shoes from Dior Homme and hat from New York.

▶ You don't see many Norfolk jackets on the streets of London these days, which is what made Calum stand out. It's a lovely smart, yet not too formal, way of wearing tweed. Love the belting detail and the large pockets, which are characteristics of the Norfolk, with this one by Oliver Spencer. Teaming it with jeans makes the look more contemporary and the folky scarf, by Waterloo Station, adds a playful touch. The 1950s-style Paul Smith frames continue the vintage feel.

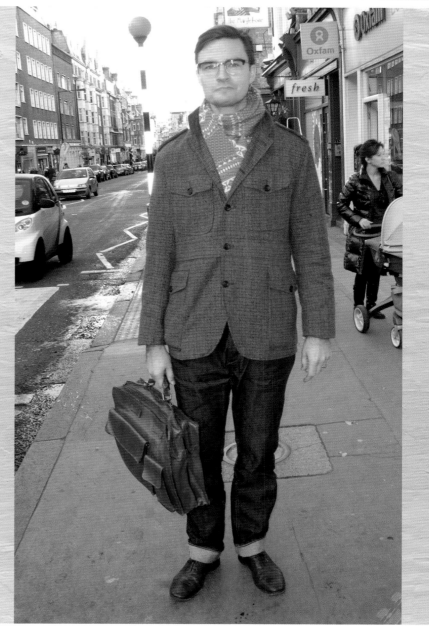

NEW YORK

◀ This is pure city slicker. The suit is lightweight but he's gone heavy on the accessories – sunglasses, tie-pin, pocket square and tote. He looks "dressed" but it works and doesn't seem too much, thanks to the brown suede shoes and blue tone-on-tones helping to keep the look grounded. If he'd worn shiny or patent shoes, it would have crossed over.

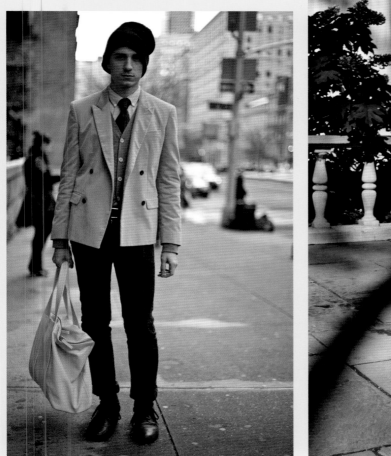

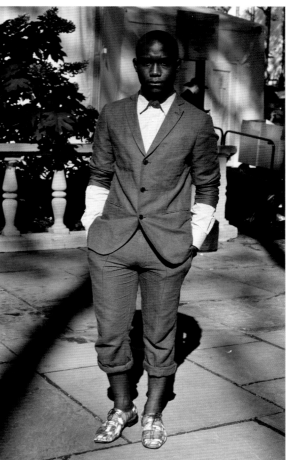

▲ Many men shy away from strong colours but the best way to carry it off is to almost ignore it. This guy looks like he's just put on a jacket that happened to be bright yellow and that's the way to play it. The rest of the outfit isn't saying "look at me" which tones the jacket down. The jacket's a nice, slightly shrunken DB cut with peaked lapels and it balances the over-large tote. The button-down Oxford shirt echoes the buttons on the cardigan, making this a great layered winter look.

▲ Summer dressing in the city is a major headache; you want to look dressed, but not die in the heat. Here is a great idea: the linen suit is thin enough to roll up the legs, the arms have been pushed up to reveal the shirt underneath and by buttoning the shirt up to the top the look retains formality. If he'd worn sandals it might have been too casual so these Madras-patterned shoes say summer without crossing over into holiday territory.

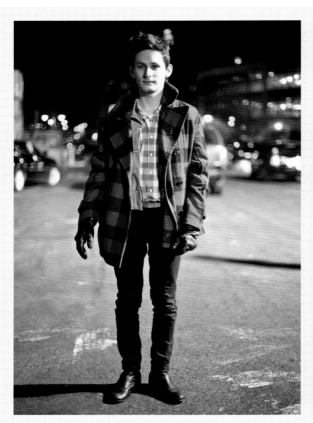

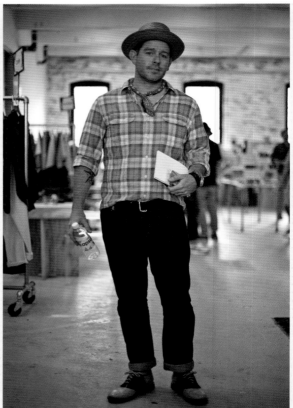

▲ This is a strong Americana look: the Buffalo check is classically bold and nicely reflects the smaller checks on the shirt. The slim jeans and boots say "workwear" in a fashion sense. All of his layers are revealed – the white T-shirt, the shirt, the jacket and the coat – giving the look depth.

▲ This is fun. He looks like a character from a Mark Twain novel. The necktie gives it a whimsical, tongue-in-cheek quality and the boater and two-tone saddle shoes continue the vintage theme. His watch and tattoo add contemporary touches, which bring the look up to date and make it cool.

▶ Double denim has been a massive trend. This guy has chosen to match the denim tones so the look almost becomes a suit. The asymmetric details on the chest pockets and detailing on the shoulder add interest while the sunglasses and hat add a good dose of cool. I like the way he rolled up the legs but not the arms, so you get to see what a great shirt it is.

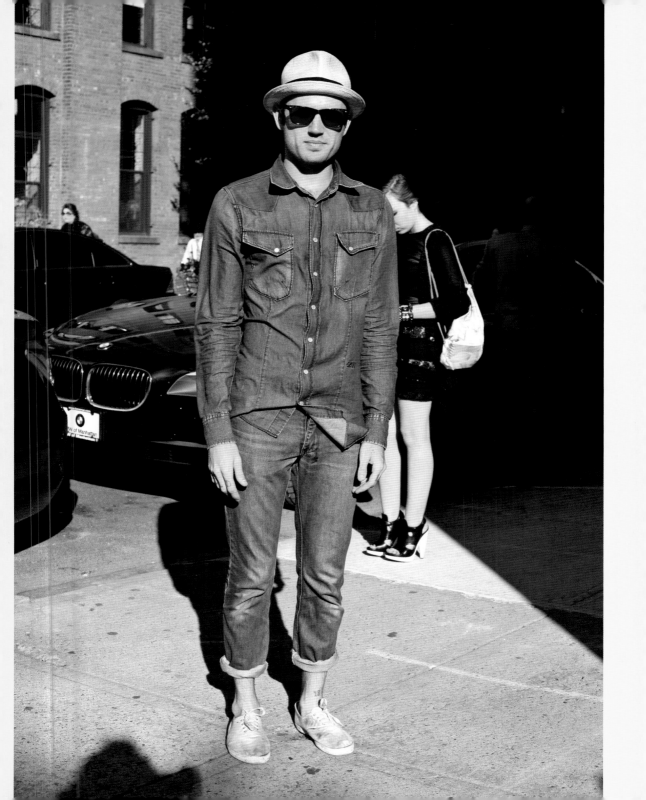

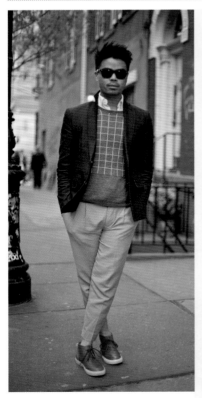

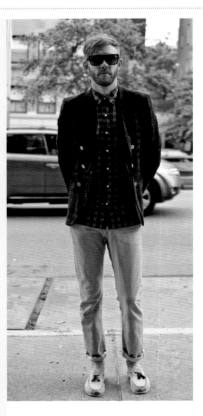

▲ Nowhere does preppy like the USA. Here we have the jacket, chinos, shirt and round-neck sweater, all components to preppy but not old-fashioned or stuffy. The box pleats on the trousers and the shrunken jacket, combined with the geometric detailing of the sweater, bring it bang up to date. Dark sunglasses add anonymity.

▲ This is "Hamptons chic". Americans are very good at combining warm weather and style. The shorts are long and wide, giving a *Great Gatsby* 1930s feel. The white driving shoes echo the shorts and the detailing on the lapel of the boating-style jacket. This guy tans well enough to get away with strong white. The necktie is the finishing smart touch.

▲ This look is all quite unstructured and could quite easily have been a bit of a mess but the tweaks and details keep it tight. The untucked shirt has a square finish, which elongates the top half and balances him out. The tassels on the shoes and gold buttons on the jacket are traditional while the severe line of the sunglasses create a contemporary contrast. Very cool.

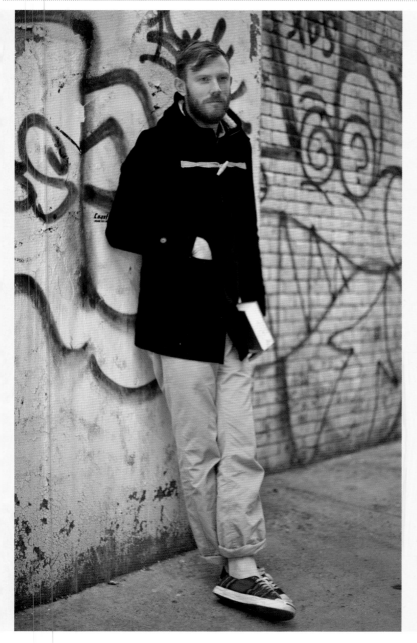

◄ This is very romantic – he could be a great American writer from the 1950s. The duffel coat is a timeless classic and with the red beard he looks like a nineteenth-century fisherman. The book, chinos and checked trainers (sneakers) add the retro collegiate vibe.

PARIS

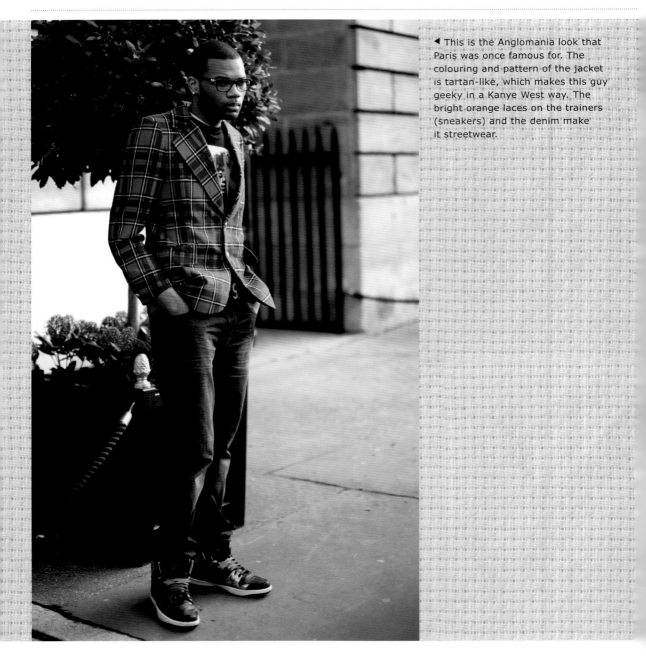

◀ This is the Anglomania look that Paris was once famous for. The colouring and pattern of the jacket is tartan-like, which makes this guy geeky in a Kanye West way. The bright orange laces on the trainers (sneakers) and the denim make it streetwear.

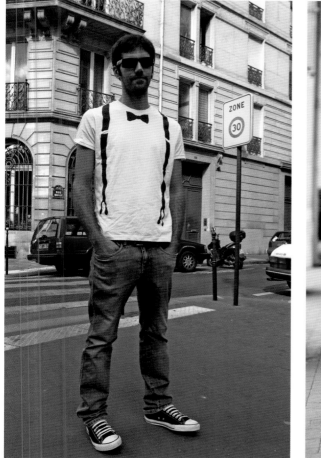

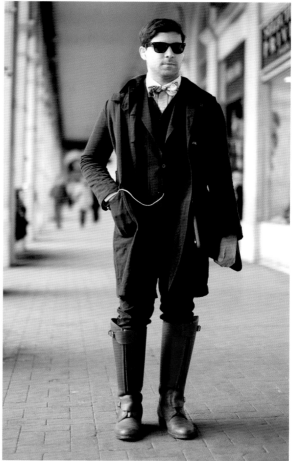

▲ Michele here is wearing a simple outfit of T-shirt, jeans and Converse. The white T-shirt is printed with a quirky trompe l'oeil design, which plays with the idea of formality, and the black bow-tie is echoed in strong-framed sunglasses.

▲ This is equestrian Paris: the city of Hermès and the art of saddlery. The boots look very solid and sturdy. It's sort of eighteenth century and then you see the Wayfarers and laptop case and it almost becomes a joke. The bow-tie is cool and the iPod wire looks like a pocket watch.

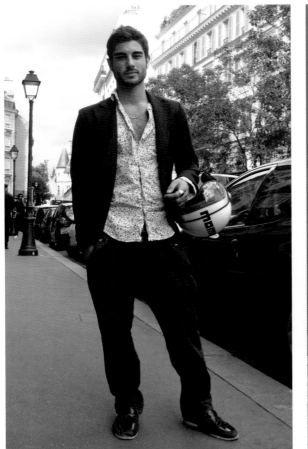

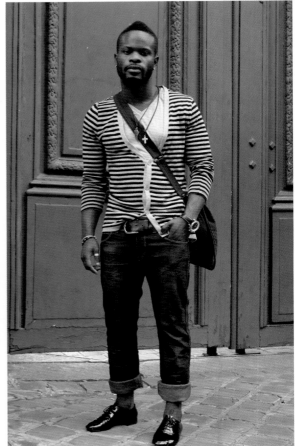

▲ Nico, here at the Hotel de Ville in Paris, looks pretty smooth but the outfit is quite interesting. His jacket is unstructured so seems to drape, the shirt is cut short so works untucked and the trousers are relaxed and wide. The proportions of this look are good and say "smartly chilled", while the patent boat shoes are a nice finishing touch. C'est bon!

▲ This would be a fairly standard outfit if it wasn't for the ankles. Like any sexy Victorian lady, the ankles should be on titillating display! Kayron, photographed in La Marais, Paris, has rolled his jeans into large cuffs and teamed them with patent lace-ups. Looks good.

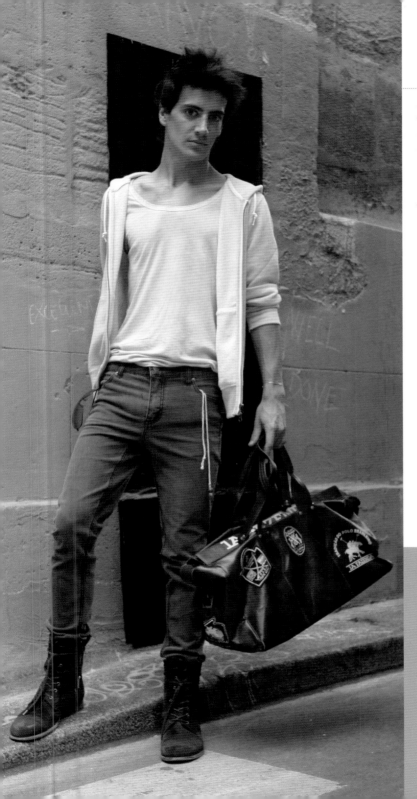

◄ This is like a fashion gym outfit. The bag looks a little D-Squared with all the badges. Grégoire's look is lean and simple: the Zara T-shirt has a wide neck which helps it drape and boxer-style boots by All Saints look best with the jeans tucked in. The jacket is by Uniqlo and the jeans are by Cheap Monday.

STOCKHOLM

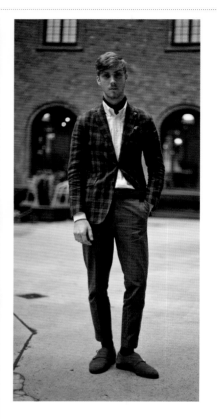

◄ Pure Swedish cool. The Scandinavians have a knack for keeping their looks so effortless and simple. This is quite Andy Warhol: the blond mop, stripy T-shirt and black jeans. A uniform of simplicity, it's relaxed, easy and body-conscious but not showy.

▲ This is so neat and clean. It's dressed but also very relaxed. I like the neckerchief, pocket square and monk-strap shoes. He looks like a young boy trying to dress up as a man, which makes it really cute. Playful.

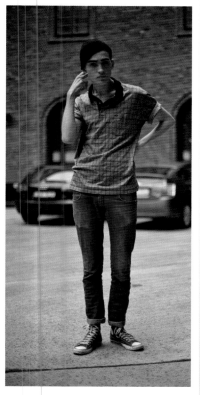

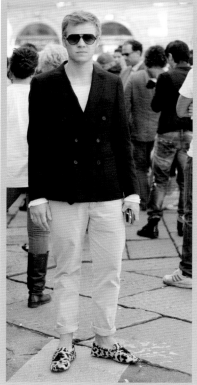

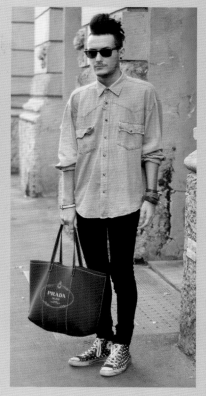

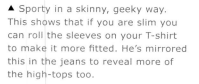

▲ Sporty in a skinny, geeky way. This shows that if you are slim you can roll the sleeves on your T-shirt to make it more fitted. He's mirrored this in the jeans to reveal more of the high-tops too.

▲ The Italians always have to have that little bit of flamboyance. This guy's outfit is a clean summer look – the double-breasted navy jacket and turned-up chinos – and then you see the sparkle of personality, the leopard-print shoes. It's sometimes good to have a touch of humour in your outfit and here he makes it work well.

▲ A play of proportions, the denim shirt is oversized while the trousers are super-skinny. The obviously designer bag is typically Italian but the necklace and bracelets add a creative and arty edge.

TOKYO

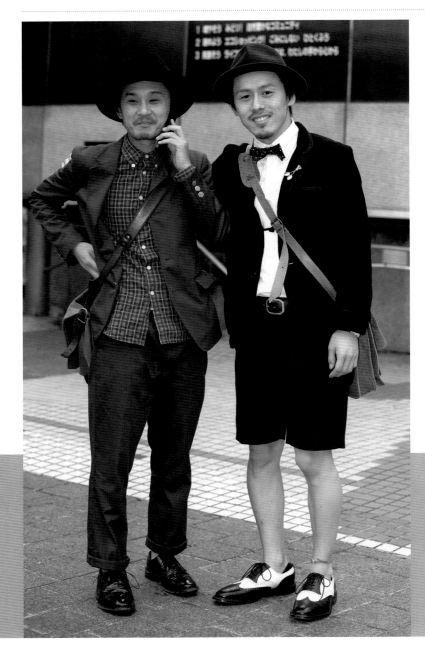

◀ The guys in Tokyo take inspiration from all over the world: a little bit of England here, America there. These two definitely have a large dose of Germany. On the right, the outfit looks like lederhosen while both hats resemble mountaineer headgear. The bags worn across the chest and the sleeve buttons and badge make them look like they are part of some Boy Scout fashion club.

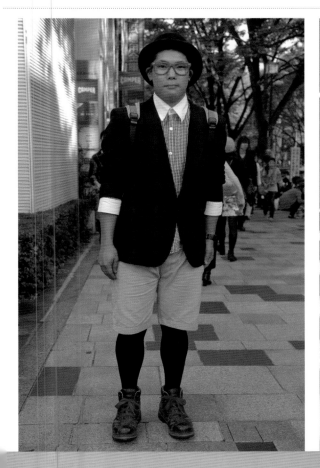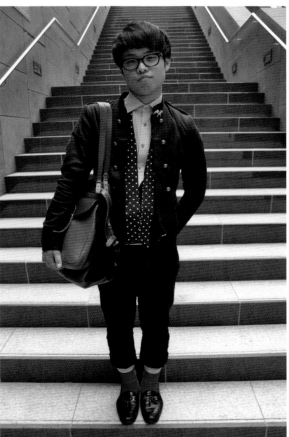

▲ Here's a look of youthful playfulness: he's a Japanese schoolboy with a backpack and shorts mixed with old-fashioned "English banker" bowler. The laces on the boots correspond with the spectacle frames, adding a flash of colour.

▲ The Japanese are very good at playing with proportions. This guy has made his top half longer by heavily cropping the trousers, revealing all of the red socks. The large bag is a deliberate attempt to shrink the rest of him.

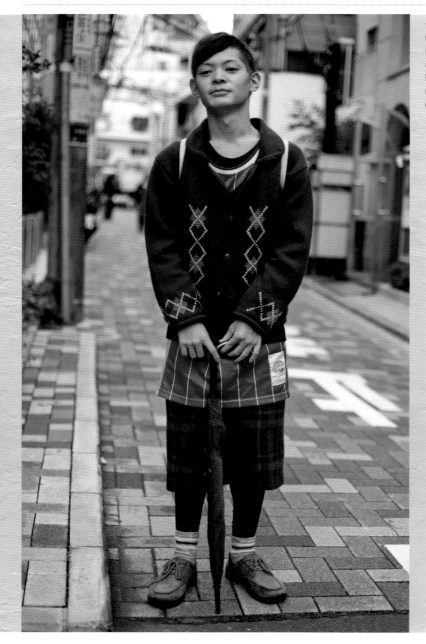

◄ Only in Japan would you see this: the guy is wearing three graduating layers. It looks almost monastic until you see the middle layer is a basketball jersey. The Japanese are masters at layering and here he has done it in a way to elongate himself.

▶ This is American preppy done the Japanese way. The Aran-style tank top with cricket detailing around the neck, gingham shirt, smart lace-up shoes and chinos are classic WASP-wear but it's the A Bathing Ape gorilla stuck on the front that gives it away as Japanese.

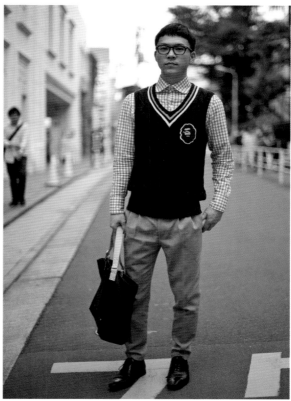

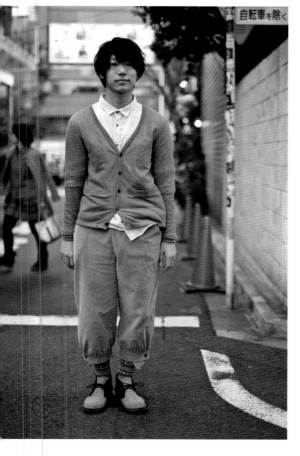

◀ This look is slightly dishevelled but in an artistic way. The trousers are like plus fours, but worn down. It all says "intellectual student" who's far too busy to care about the frivolities of dress, yet comes out looking extremely cool.

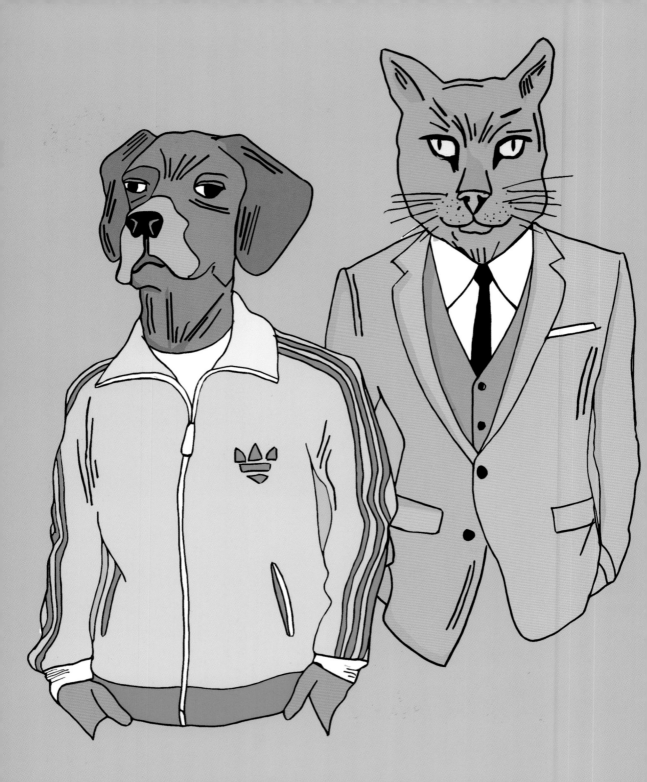

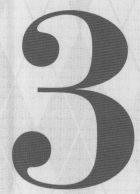

Fashion for the Geek

This is where the magic happens. Your wardrobe is the all-encompassing expression of your style. Think of it as your own personal archive to which you keep adding; a mix of designer, vintage, high street, even charity finds, which will provide the finest array of choice. The modern man's wardrobe should contain many different departments for all the occasions and places in his professional and social diaries. A tasteful and varied wardrobe will make getting dressed and looking good a whole lot easier. This section will help you identify what is available and give you a little guidance on each area.

To simplify getting dressed, think of it as a bit like cooking; use a well-chosen set of ingredients in a certain way to achieve the required result. Style is a mix of different things which, like a recipe, have to be used in the right amounts. Some can judge this by eye while others need a step-by-step guide. Think of some outfits as snacks and others as more complicated Michelin-starred dishes.

★ Always start with good-quality ingredients.

★ Crack basic recipes first and then work your way up to more complicated ones.

★ Once you've perfected a look, you can start playing around and throw your own touches into the mix.

★ Have a varied diet. Try new things.

★ Stop when things can get too fussy. Sometimes all you'll want is the sartorial equivalent of beans on toast.

★ You can easily overcook it; watch what you're doing at each stage.

★ Taste! You are now ready to be served. Voilà, Style!

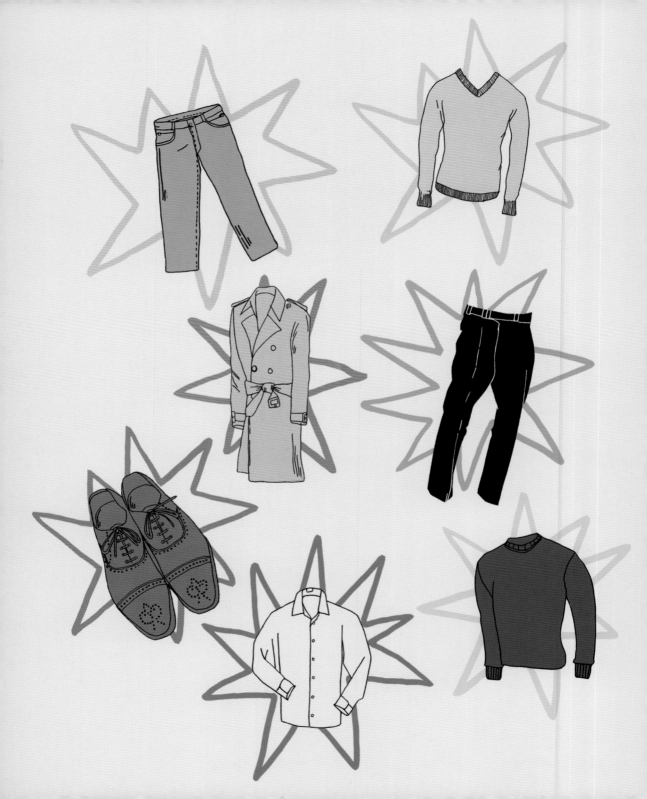

Creating a Capsule Wardrobe

Mastering the capsule wardrobe will make getting dressed in the morning easy, as it is the framework on which to build the rest of your wardrobe. Stick to The Chic Geek's list of items and you really can't go wrong. The majority of pieces will work with each other in various combinations and have you looking subtly stylish from day to night, every day.

Getting these basics right is the foundation to being stylish. Think of them like ingredients in a kitchen – the salt and pepper or ketchup of men's style!

Most of the items recommended are navy, grey or white; these colours are masculine, clean, suit nearly everybody and look great in our climate. Try to buy the best quality you can afford and make sure the fit is good, then nobody will be able to fault you. Avoid slogans or logos – think plain and tasteful.

White Shirt The simplest item but probably one of the hardest to find and get right. There are so many details and variations it may take a while to find the perfect one for you. When you do, buy lots.

Black Oxfords Think the best school shoes you've ever had.

Trenchcoat Stay away from the traditional beige, which looks a bit dated, and go for navy or another darker colour. This will be your wet weather mainstay.

Black Trousers This is your formal piece; if in doubt you can always chuck on a pair of slim black trousers.

Grey V-neck Sweater The depth of the "V" changes due to fashion, but the grey V-neck never goes away.

Brown Brogues Classic round-toe English-style brogues get better and better with time.

Black and Brown Belts Keep the buckles to a minimum and not too flashy.

Camel Three-button Formal Overcoat No matter how hot you think you look, you'll still need to keep warm!

White Polo Shirt The freshest and cleanest colour, which looks pure and innocent!

Grey, Navy and White Plain Crewneck T-shirts Buy thin cotton or a synthetic mix, which show off the body better.

Blue Jeans Straight or slim leg fit in a dark blue wash.

White Underwear Never dates, looks clean and doesn't fade or age as much as coloured underwear.

Coloured Socks Preferably striped and bold. Plain socks just look a little "old-man" unless they're black (but even these are better with coloured toes or tops).

Navy Wool Two-button Suit A classic, this will work anywhere. You can always wear the jacket separately if you get a short one, and the trousers may be worn with any of knitwear.

Navy Cardigan Versatile and can be worn open or buttoned.

Navy Round-neck Sweater Simple shape, deep rich colour and worn with jeans – perfect. Choose cashmere, preferably, as it will hold the deep colour much better.

Seasonal Touches

Let's talk about the two extremes of the year: heat and cold. Unfortunately in the northern hemisphere there's usually a lot more cold than heat, so The Chic Geek's advice is to get yourself a large plastic storage box with a lid – very important – and store one season's wardrobe while the other is out and then swap when needs must.

In summer the box will store all those "extreme cold" favourites such as gloves, fur hats, scarves, winter boots, tweeds, etc. The lid will prevent moths or anything spoiling those precious items. In winter the box will contain sandals, sunglasses, beach items, summer shirts, shorts, linen hats, etc.

As well as being a good way to care for your clothes, using storage boxes will clear space in your wardrobe or bedroom and keep everything together; often you forget what you own, so you will be pleasantly surprised when you open the box. It feels like a shopping trip without the expense.

Trousers

Slacks, strides, pants, call them what you will, trousers are usually a tailored item with belt loops and a fly front. They were the most masculine item of male dress until women got in the act during the twentieth century. There are two choices today for a man to wear below the waist: denim jeans or trousers. Here are the different types that fit in the "trouser" box.

Styles

Checked Trousers These are a bold choice – very Rupert the Bear – and range from a tasteful Prince of Wales check to a bold tartan. When wearing them, balance the bold with a plain top.

Chinos The chino sits nicely between denim jeans and formal trousers. If jeans are too casual and formal trousers too dressy, chinos are the balance between the two. They are simple cotton trousers in a dusty or earth colour that is also known as "khaki".

Corduroy The wale is the thickness of the cord. Corduroy comes in a multitude of wales, from thin to jumbo, depending on how refined you want to be. Corduroys are a classic of English dress, particularly the brightly coloured reds, greens and corn.

Jean Styles The five-pocket jean style is synonymous with denim, but this style comes in a multitude of other fabrics, such as corduroy or moleskin for a more casual look.

Moleskin This fabric has the soft and smooth feel of a mole. Hardwearing, this trouser is another traditional classic alongside corduroys and comes in the same rainbow of bold colours.

Tuxedo Trousers These are usually black and worn to formal events. Easy to identify, they have a satin strip of material that runs down the outside of both legs. Tuxedo trousers are usually made of a luxurious blend of wool and mohair.

Velvet An evening-dress fabric that can be worn instead of tuxedo trousers with a velvet dinner jacket. Velvet trousers look good under subdued lighting and in rich jewel colours.

Wool This is the traditional material for formal trousers. There are different mixes, depending on the quality and price of the trouser.

Details

Turn-ups A turn-up (also called a "cuff") is where the material has been turned outward to form a band at the bottom of the trouser – the size of these is a personal choice. Turn-ups help in two ways: they protect and add weight to the trouser hem so the drape of the trouser is better. If you are short, turn-ups can make your legs look shorter so they are best avoided. Turn-ups give an old-fashioned formality and a nice detail to the bottom of the leg, especially to a wide-legged trouser.

Pleats These are the folds at the front of the trouser of which you can have as many as you like, but usually one, two or three. A pleat that opens toward the pocket is called a reverse pleat and a pleat that opens toward the zip is known as a forward pleat. The more pleats you have, the more dramatic it looks from the front, but this can make the rear suffer so your derrière disappears.

Flat Fronted This is a type of trouser without pleats.

Side Adjusters Most trousers have belt loops so you can add a belt for support, but some trousers do away with this by having side adjusters that, when pulled tight, make the trousers fit perfectly on the waist.

Fly The fly is the covering of the fastening of the trouser. There are usually two options: a zip or button fly.

Jeans

Denim jeans have become the default trouser – if in doubt, throw on a pair of jeans. Suitable for everything apart from weddings and funerals, the denim jean is something you should spend the most time in finding the correct shape and style. The denim jean has over the years come in every shape or treatment imaginable.

Cuts

Bootcut The bootcut sits low on the hips, is slim through the thigh and then has a slight flare from knee to ankle to cover the shoe or boot.

Flare A style that is similar to bootcut but much more exaggerated. This style hasn't been around for many years but will, no doubt, return.

Skinny This is the style du jour but unfortunately it does exclude some people. If you have big thighs this is a no – they should be fitted, not skintight. The skinny looks good on the shoe, cut slightly short or turned up to reveal the sock. Always look for a bit of stretch in the material, as this will help it keep its shape better and the jean will be more comfortable to wear.

Slim This style fits close through the backside and thigh through to the ankle where it is slightly tapered. These jeans do not have much loose fabric, so if you want the skinny look but not too severe, this is a good style.

Straight This jean fits straight through the leg, neither tight nor loose. It's a classic-looking jean that generally sits higher on the waist.

Denim Jean Tips

★ Any colour is good but you can never go wrong with a deep inky blue.

★ Your backside should look good; if it doesn't try another pair.

★ No zips or dangly things, especially on the back pockets.

★ Go easy on the branding. You should be paid to be a walking billboard.

★ Keep your jeans quite plain with no designs or tattooing on the denim.

★ Go easy on the distressing, rips or tears. Jeans should look naturally aged.

★ Bleached denim is a certainly "a look" – and one to avoid.

★ Skinny jeans should not be so tight that they look like they are painted on.

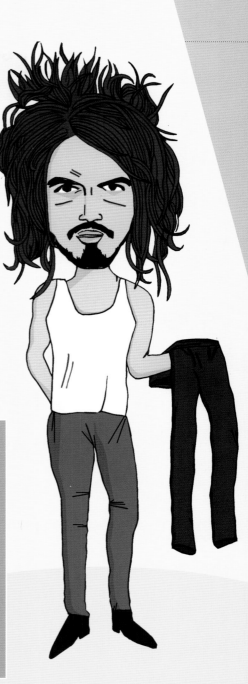

Formal Shirts

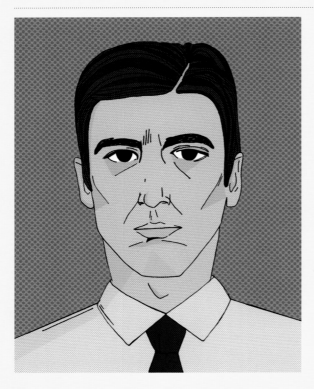

It is surprising how many details there are in a simply shirt and how many choices and options you have. From fabric to cut to collars to cuffs, the variations are endless. The formal shirt has had a rough time of it of late, looking a little old-fashioned, but it is still something we need to own. Whatever style you choose, never, ever wear a formal shirt untucked.

Most retailers now offer a slim-cut shirt, which rids the shirt of all that unsightly excess material on the sides and has you feeling less like you're wearing your dad's clothes. Shirts should fit well on the shoulder and neck and you want the overall fit to be not too tight – you have to be able to move and be comfortable.

Choose simple, button-down cuffs. On some shirts there will be different button widths to allow for your watch, which is a nice touch. Double or French cuffs haven't been cool for a while but in the right formal environment they can work. Double cuffs can be too fiddly if you're in a rush as you need cufflinks, and they get much dirtier than regular button-down cuffs.

Collar Shapes

There are a lot of collar shapes and some designers or brands have their own signature cut or angle to the collar.

Turndown Collars These collars are the traditional shape with the tips of the collar pointing downward and the size should be in proportion to your neck and body. Collars have been getting smaller of late – the large collar is a little too "city boy" – but the size has to allow for the option of a necktie.

Spread or Cutaway Collars The wider opening at the front shows off the necktie better and the tips point to the side. This is the style often seen on Italian men and is associated with Italian brands.

Round or Club Collar A rounded collar, this style has no tips, so only works on a thinner collar. It looks cool in a 1920s working-class way.

Tab Collar A small buttoned tab connects the collars behind the necktie, thus pushing it forward. You don't see this style very often, but it is a nice novelty and looks very dapper and neat.

Wing Collars Only for dinner dress, the wing is used to accommodate a bow tie.

Button-down Collar This can be a little too casual for some, but worn with a necktie it oozes preppy cool and holds the tie nicely in place.

Placket Though not a collar shape, it is important to know this term. The placket is the part of the shirt where the collar meets the front opening and where the buttons are. On a concealed placket, the buttons are covered, which is great for a streamlined, minimal look, and is a feature often found on dress shirts.

T-shirt Advice

Once only an undergarment, the T-shirt or "tee" has become an excuse to show off all those hours spent in the gym. One of the simplest items in a man's wardrobe, it can also be the most difficult to track down when looking for the perfect and most flattering T-shirt in terms of cut and material. The most ubiquitous item a man owns, the humble tee has become dangerously disposable. Find one that works for you and stick to it. Here is The Chic Geek's T-shirt advice.

★ Keep it simple. The T-shirt should be a basic layer, whether worn on its own or with other items.

★ The T-shirt should drape; it should be fitted but not skintight.

★ Choose a material with a bit of stretch. This will help the T-shirt to keep its shape and cling better.

★ If you are skinny and don't have the natural "guns", roll the sleeves to avoid that telltale, pointy-out triangle on the arms.

★ Male cleavage or "heavage" is getting out of control; no deep Vs or gratuitous displays of flesh, please. Less is more.

★ It is fine to deviate from the norm. The Henley is a round neck with buttons down the front; the polo shirt is like a Henley but with a collar and a shorter cap sleeve to reveal more bicep – very '50s Marlon Brando.

★ Turn the volume down on the designs and colour; subtle is stylish.

★ From Katherine Hamnett to Henry Holland, the slogan T-shirt rears its ugly head every now and again. Try to avoid.

★ When you find a T-shirt that you like and that works for you, multiple buy.

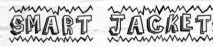

SMART JACKETS

The traditional sports jacket was originally
an item worn by the wealthy while hunting,
shooting and fishing in the countryside. When
we speak about modern sportswear, this is not
something that usually comes to mind and is
now considered smart casual dress. Basically a
tailored jacket, the sports jacket is a suit jacket
that isn't worn with matching trousers.

Blazer The blazer had a bad name because
of the "gin-and-jag" brigade but has recently
become a retro, cool item. Choose a cropped
body. Traditionally these were made in navy
wool and were double-breasted with the
signature gold buttons.

Corduroy Jacket Another hardwearing
country fabric, the corduroy jacket is
synonymous with the university professor
and looks great with the ironic elbow patches.

Tweed Jacket This is the classic sports jacket
made in hundreds of different colours, designs
and weights of tweed. It is something that will
last a lifetime and moulds to your body in time.
Looks good with a matching waistcoat.

Velvet Smoking Jacket A character piece,
this resembles a velvet jacket but has a shawl
collar, quilting and extra detailing on the front.
An evening item that is definitely to be worn
tongue-in-cheek.

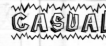
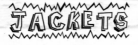

Jackets are items that usually end at or just below the waist. Here is a rundown of the casual favourites.

Anorak A synthetic waterproof jacket with a hood. More practical than stylish, this jacket is good for festivals and the great outdoors.

Biker Jacket This is a leather jacket with asymmetric zips on the front. It should be worn tight and made of the thinnest and most supple leather you can afford. Rick Owens has built a whole brand on this jacket.

Bomber Jacket A treasured item of the skin-heads, it still has the same connotations. A thin, round-necked jacket originally made for pilots.

Blouson This is a cropped jacket with a wide ribbed band at the bottom and on the cuffs. It looks chic with smart trousers and makes you seem tall.

Collegiate or Baseball Jacket A preppy home run, this is similar to a bomber with its round neck. Look for jackets with the towelling letters and team details and wear very fitted.

Donkey Jacket This is a short, workman's jacket that has the protective panels over the shoulders. Choose one with subtle detailing – definitely no high-vis!

Harrington The Baracuta G9, as it is otherwise known, is a neat, zip-front, tartan-lined jacket often associated with Steve McQueen and skinheads. Suits everybody.

Jean Jacket An American classic and the more beat-up, the better. Wear fitted and don't be afraid to mix different coloured denims.

Waxed Jacket A coated jacket to keep you dry. Look for plenty of nice details: pockets, checked linings, etc. The Barbour is the go-to brand for a classic waxed jacket.

The Suit

The male suit is a man's uniform; basically it's a smart jacket with matching trousers. For centuries the suit has clothed the male gentleman and continues to do so because a good suit will have you looking taller, slimmer, sexier and more elegant.

Worn to work, formal functions or just for the sheer hell of it, over the years the suit has continually evolved to reflect the fashions of the day. The shapes and styles that this 3.5 metres (nearly 4 yards) of fabric can be tailored into are never-ending and, as such, it is the most chronicled of male dress.

The standard modern lounge suit is usually a fitted, single-breasted jacket with two or three buttons in a sombre colour and matching flat-fronted trousers. Jacket lengths have become shorter (thanks to designers such as Thom Browne who have pushed a shrunken silhouette) and trousers have become slimmer. This style of suit would stand any man in good stead. There are, of course, many other options. Here is The Chic Geek's advice on ready-to-wear suits.

★ Fit is so important. The suit needs to sit well on the body and finish to the right lengths on the arms and legs. Forget the brand name or price, it's all about the fit.

★ Try different styles and sizes, get an idea about what you like and what fits your body best.

★ If the suit is a work suit and has a job to do, make sure the fabric will withstand the rigours of this. Buy a spare pair of trousers as these will wear out more quickly than the jacket.

★ Never button the last button of the jacket as generally it looks a bit uptight if you do. Edward VII was said to have started this trend because of his large girth.

★ Double-breasted suits generally look better on taller guys.

★ You might like to turn the suit from a two-piece into a three-piece by adding a waistcoat, if the option is there, which creates a neater look. The waistcoat works especially well in traditional fabrics such as tweed and Prince of Wales check.

★ The big rule: you wear the suit, never let the suit wear you.

★ Avoid fancy, garish-coloured linings.

The Bespoke Suit

The bespoke suit is the haute couture of menswear. This is where you have carte blanche over style and material. You choose everything from scratch; the width of the lapel, pockets, buttons, linings, vents, the list goes on. It can be overwhelming at first with the amount of choices and decisions to be made but this is a male sartorial rite of passage and as such is a very special experience. If you are thinking of having a bespoke suit made, consider the following advice.

★ Don't rush into anything; this is a big investment. Look at other suits you own or have seen that you like and make a mental note of the elements you like about them.

★ Tailors have their own house style so do some research and see which ones you like. The best in the world are on London's Savile Row where the suits are hand-stitched using traditional techniques. Savile Row can seem quite a daunting place but remember there is a first time for everyone.

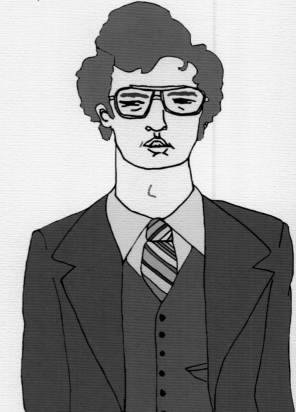

★ Speak to the tailor, see what they recommend. They've had more experience than you and also know what is possible.

★ Take a picture from a magazine or any other inspirational material as this will help them to understand exactly what you want and expect.

★ What do you want this suit to say and do? Should it earn its keep or is it for a special occasion?

★ Don't be afraid to say you don't like something at any stage. You should never be disappointed.

★ Follow the Duke of Windsor's example: wear bespoke forever and if your body changes then the suit can always be altered.

★ Your bespoke suit is the only one in the world. Your name and the month and year it was made are written inside the pocket. Nobody else has this; it's a very special thing.

How to Choose a Suit

The advice below is given by **Patrick Grant of Norton & Sons**, one of Savile Row's finest bespoke tailors. Established in 1821, the house made its name tailoring to the young and sporting among Europe's elite.

The firm gained eminence making sharply cut suits for rugged and robust gentlemen, such as Lord Mountbatten and the young Winston Churchill, for whom they made everything from dinner suits to racing silks. Lord Carnarvon wore a Norton suit when he discovered Tutankhamun's tomb. Norton & Sons still hand-cuts and hand-sews every garment on Savile Row, using the traditional techniques perfected over centuries of tailoring. A well-fitting suit of classical proportions in simple cloth forms the foundation of a good wardrobe. An English bespoke tailor will cut you a good suit. If your suit is to last you 20 years, it is best to avoid fad or fashion. There are three simple rules.

① Buy few suits but good suits.

② Favour simple suiting but splendid linen.

③ Always let one's clothes be correct, never too formal nor too casual, never too worn nor too new.

"I favour a single-breasted two-button jacket with a notched lapel, straight pockets and side vents, and a higher cut flat-fronted trouser. If your finances allow, start with the following: dark navy flannel, dark charcoal flannel, navy worsted, charcoal worsted, Glenurquhart check worsted, navy cable stripe worsted. For warmer days add a couple of frescos, again in navy and charcoal.

"Armed with his simple suits a gentleman can set forth to create his look with shirtings and silks as simply or as flamboyantly as his tastes allow. It is with his linens that an Englishman expresses his sense of dress. One's shirts must be well-cut and should be classically proportioned. Experiment until you find a collar shape that works. A good shirtmaker will assist in your choice of cut and guide you through the many thousand cotton shirtings and tie silks that he will offer. And one should neither overdress nor underdress. Dress for the occasion and avoid looking contrived. According to the wonderful George Frazier, 'No well-dressed man's clothes should look either old or new.'

"I wear a dinner suit of my grandfather's, cut in 1936, which age and wear has rendered perfect. The Norton & Son's suit that I wear today I have worn at least 100 times before. It took about 50 wears before it really felt worn in. Purchasers of inexpensive suits will never experience this joy."

How to Have a Bespoke Suit Made

English tailor **Henry Herbert** shows The Chic Geek how to have a bespoke suit made. Sir Henry Herbert was master of the royal wardrobe to both King Charles I and King Charles II, responsible for their tunicae and viseres (shirts and hats). Charlie Collingwood resurrected the Henry Herbert name when he established his tailors, who use a fleet of Vespas to visit and measure up customers throughout London. Carrying tape measures, chalk and the finest selection of wools, linens and silks from the UK's most traditional and long-established mills, Henry Herbert tailors will come to you whenever and wherever to measure up and make up perfectly fitting handmade suits.

Part 1: Meeting the Tailor

This is the first part of having a bespoke suit made – the initial consultation, measuring and deciding on style and fabric. At this point you can, within reason, have whatever you want – any fabric, lining, shape, buttons, pockets, lapels, finish and detailing.

The first decision is fabric; this influences everything else. The Chic Geek chose a brown pepper-and-salt Donegal tweed by Porter & Harding, a mill in Exeter, for his suit. The next decision is shape: single- or double-breasted. Then comes choosing one, two, three or four buttons on the suit. The number of decisions can be daunting but a good tailor will advise according to a customer's body shape. The Chic Geek chose a simple two-button single-breasted suit, which is quite humble. Because subtly is the key, a notched lapel and one cut at the back was chosen. Then lining was discussed and a dark brown lining by Dugdale Brothers in Huddersfield, Yorkshire, was selected.

Finally measurements are taken. The whole process should take around an hour and at the end you are given a card with a sample of the suit and lining fabric. An appointment is arranged for four weeks time when a initial mock-up of the suit will be ready to try on.

Part 2: The First Try On

This is the exciting part: the cloth has been cut and you get to see the suit for first time. First you try on the trousers to make sure the waist is comfortable and then you sit up and down to ensure the "seat" is good and allows you sit without the trousers becoming too tight on the legs. You also look at the length and width of the trousers. If you don't like anything or feel uncomfortable, this is your chance to speak up.

The jacket is unlined and at this stage everything can be adjusted. For example, on The Chic Geek's suit, the shoulders needed to be narrowed and the bottom of the jacket had to be curved. Because the shoulders were being narrowed, the lapels needed to be made smaller. Suits are all about proportions; if you change one aspect, this has a knock-on effect in other areas.

Every area is examined, noting for example how the pockets slant, where the buttons are to be placed and the arm length. Once you are happy, the suit is taken away to be finished.

Part 3: The Finished Suit

The suit is finally finished. All the waiting is over and the expectation is high. You try it on for the final time, with all the alterations from the previous meeting completed, and the last thing the tailor does is cut open the buttonholes. There you have it: one amazing bespoke suit. The great thing about bespoke is you're walking around in one of kind – nobody has this suit because it was made just for you.

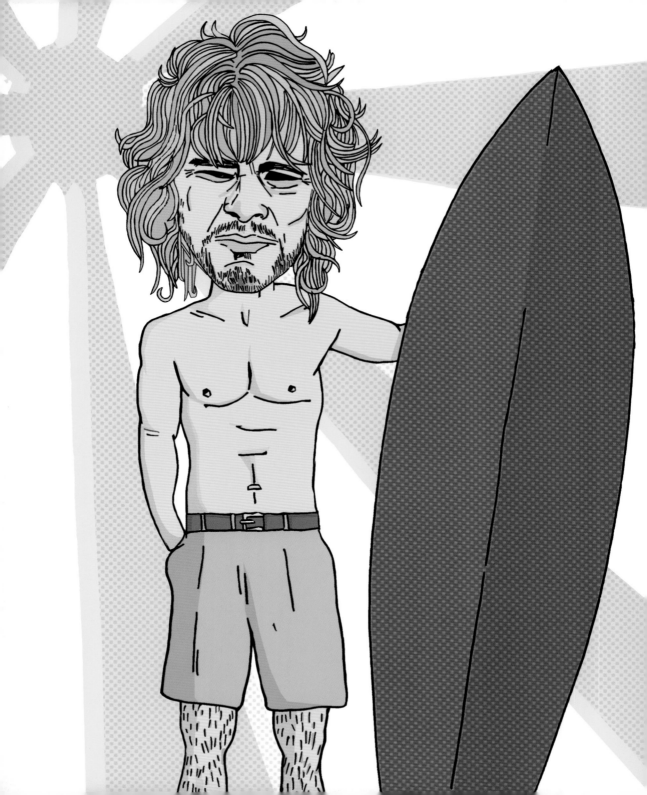

Sportswear

Let's talk sports. Aesthetically you want to sit somewhere between professional and amateur. Sometimes it all depends on how good you are but nobody needs it rubbed in their faces, and all the bells and whistles equipment can have you looking a little try-hard. Best to be a bit coy about your abilities.

Gym Stick to a combination of tones of the same colours, preferably dark, so everything works together. Wear only subtle logos and no slogans; keep it clean and slick so even when you are sweating you still look together.

Designer clothes at the gym can seem a little wrong or showy, so keep it simple and understated. Save the body for the showers so nothing too clingy or revealing. Leave the oversized "Golds Gym" wife-beaters to the dumb-bells in the corner.

Swimming When you swim you have to think about the journey into the water. This is the bit where you are seen, the walk from the changing rooms to the pool. How do you want to look? You should want to go unnoticed, unless you're Michael Phelps. Even if you have a bod to die for, a stylish man plays it down, so nothing too revealing or body-conscious; this is a family pool after all.

On a style note, traditional Speedos do look a little dated and the tight trunk style can leave you looking top-heavy. If you want technical, "Jammers" or cycle-short styles are best for the body's proportions. For the rest of us who just want to do a few lengths, stick to loose swim shorts in a plain colour to the mid-thigh; they do drag a bit but are the perfect middle ground. Leave the bold Hibiscus prints for holidays. Goggles are acceptable, swimming caps are not.

Tennis One of the world's chicest sports: the green lawn, the crisp tennis whites and strawberries. Tennis is a social scene, so you want to go seemlessly from court to bar. Think pure white; polo shirts with a subtle monogram, white shorts to mid-thigh and white socks and trainers (sneakers). Things should be fitted but not tight. This is the only time a stylish man will be seen in white socks. You could drape a white tennis sweater over your shoulders for a touch of irony but definitely leave the head- and sweatbands to Björn Borg.

Football (Soccer) A sport of synthetics and that's just the wives and girlfriends! This is the only place for polyester.

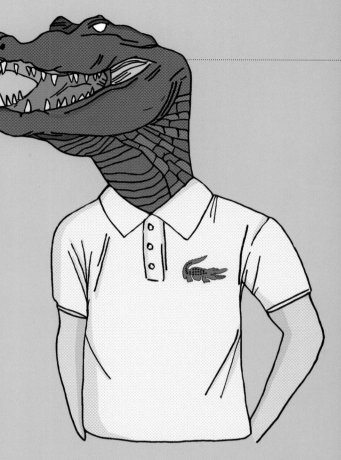

Football can be as rough and ready as the outfit; anything goes as it will soon be covered in mud and grass stains. Just don't copy professional footballer's haircuts.

Yoga You're a modern man so a spot of yoga is called for. Yoga is the "trendy" way to keep healthy and because it's fashionable, you'll want to look the part while you're swigging that wheatgrass and rolling your mat under your arm.

Wear something loose, but not hippie loose, and similar to what you would wear to the gym. This form of exercise is about tone and stretch, which is perfect because you will glow and not sweat (well, that's if you're not doing steamy Bikram yoga). Wear tracksuit bottoms if you're not very good and then move on to shorts when you want to prove your legs are straight!

Knitwear

Modern knitwear is all about luxury. Gone are the days when we would put up with something itchy or scratchy: cashmere, merino wool and silk are now the materials of choice. Although a very versatile section of your wardrobe, knitwear can also be high maintenance. Split into two camps – the fine-gauge knits, which are very elegant, and the chunky knits, thickly crafted, here's The Chic Geek's advice on knitwear.

★ If you buy cheaper knitwear, expect to have to replenish it often. This stuff won't last more than two washes.

★ Holes add character, so darn your favourites. This is part of the "shabby chic" DNA.

★ Cashmere is the best for strong colour, as it has intensity like an Anish Kapoor sculpture. Choose bold colours and avoid anything wishy-washy.

★ If you buy expensive knitwear expect to spend time hand-washing; never trust a machine with your expensive purchases.

★ When washing fine knits, turn them inside out to protect the outer surface.

★ When drying hand-washed knitwear, re-shape and dry flat, so as not to stretch the item.

★ With the big, chunky knits it is best not to wash them at all, so always wear something between your body and the knit. Dab off any stains.

★ Fine knits should be made from merino wool or another superfine quality wool or cotton that will cling to the body and look good when worn instead of a T-shirt.

★ There are classic patterns like Fair Isle, which is twee and cute, or zigzagging Missoni, which shows you've spent the money, but generally avoid pieces with too much patterning in different colours.

★ Chunky knits should be hand-knitted in traditional designs, preferably by an old Scottish or Irish lady!

★ As for styles, the cardigan is still going strong. Avoid shawl necks or anything with buckle fastenings.

Underwear

Just because people can't see it doesn't make it any less important. Underwear says a lot about you as a man and, as such, should never be an afterthought. It's a personal preference, but here are a few definite dos and don'ts.

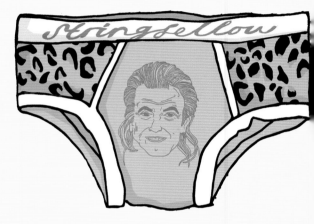

★ Acceptable underwear is underpants, trunks or boxer shorts, never thongs – this goes against everything it means to be a man.

★ Your underwear should be in proportion to your shape. If you are slim, wear a smaller piece of underwear and the reverse applies if larger.

★ Make sure your underwear fits properly and comfortably. If too tight, it will leave marks, and if too baggy, you'll look like you're wearing a nappy (diaper).

★ Stick to white, which always looks cleaner. Coloured underwear fades badly. When the white starts to discolour, replace.

★ No jokey underwear; leave the cartoons and one-liners to television.

★ There is a big trend in male control underwear for guys. If you feel this is a must, go for the most subtle pair you can find and make sure you can get them on and off in a gentlemanly fashion.

Socks

★ There are lots of "enhancement" pants available. What happened to the George Michael shuttlecock? Most of this is psychological, as once your trousers go on you'll probably not notice much difference.

★ Most underwear is hipster shape these days, which means it sits on the hips and suits the jeans we wear. Nothing is worse than those giant, apple-catcher pants that go up to the navel.

★ It is fine to have a name or logo on your underwear, but it shouldn't be visible above your trousers.

★ When you find the perfect pair, repeat buy. It looks good to have a drawerful of the same style.

Socks are to men what lingerie is to women. They are very important and, believe it or not, can make or break a whole outfit. Getting the socks right says you are a man of confidence and style. Never be afraid of colour – bold stripes or blocks add a flash of excitement between the trouser and the shoe. If wearing dark dinner shoes, stick to black, but for all other times it's carte blanche. Find a quirky balance. For example, a grey sock with a fuchsia pink pinstripe looks very chic with a suit. You get the idea.

★ DO mend any holes. Do your bit for the planet and your wallet and darn your socks with a few stitches.

★ DON'T wear cartoon, joke or novelty socks. They're just not funny, ever.

★ DO make sure the socks are long enough so that when you sit down you can't see any bare skin between sock and trouser.

★ DON'T pair thick, white sports socks with formal shoes. White socks can make a "mod" statement, but can be tricky to pull off. White tennis socks are only for trainers (sneakers) or sports shoes.

★ DO choose fabrics in wool or cashmere in winter and cotton in summer.

★ DO abide by the summer no-socks rule, which applies to sandals, boat shoes and loafers only.

★ DON'T choose logo socks. There is nothing worse than a brand name written in the sock material; the name always looks pixelated and cheap.

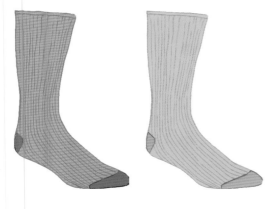

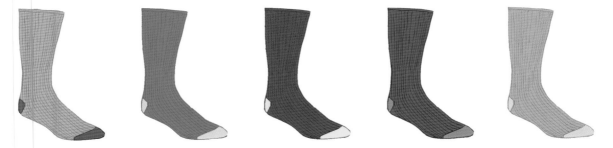

Ties, Belts & Braces

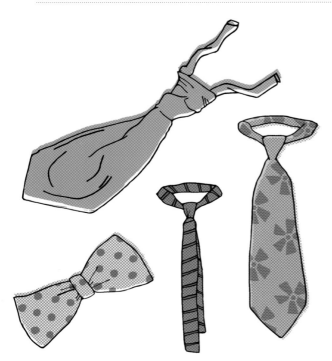

Necktie The necktie has become rather slender of late but has bounced back from super skinny and is sitting firmly at slim. It's not as showy as it once was and has spurned shiny silks for knitted or wool weaves in plain block colours. When wearing, always keep the knot small and neat and finish the tie with the tip on the waistband – the established perfect length. Only tuck it in if you're wearing it under a sweater. The necktie can compliment or contrast with your outfit but shouldn't overpower it. For patterns, club stripes are good; if unsure play safe.

Bow-ties The bow-tie works in two distinct and different ways. For night there is the O.T.T. Tom Ford dressy version in velvet, which requires something quite big and flouncy and needs a high-voltage evening outfit to go with it. On the other hand there is the day bow-tie; think neat, precise and smaller. This is *Antiques Roadshow* chic and works well in a single tone, which compliments the shirt and the rest of the outfit. Be careful with bow-ties as they can look a bit forced, so choose your moments.

Cravats This is a difficult one. Because the tie has become so much smaller, the big voluptuous cravat looks wrong at the moment. If you can find a way of making the cravat seem casual – and this will depend on fabric and pattern – then try it but generally one to avoid.

Ties

Neck decoration, be it necktie, bow-tie or cravat, should be listed on the endangered list as it's dying out. For this very reason it's interesting and standout to become involved. The amount of styles, particularly in neckties, is endless. Your choice when it comes to the different patterns, colours, textures and shapes offers an insight into your character. So best make it good. The label just denotes quality not taste or style. Hermès still make some bad ties.

The showy, shiny, silk variety now looks dated and is being replaced by matt, knitted or wool types in tasteful colours. It should blend with your suit, not shout from the middle. Note that some thick, chunky ties will never tie properly with the required small knot and will look bulbous. Never wear jokey ties, especially the ones with LEDs or batteries, even as a dare.

Belts

It's amazing how something as simple as a belt, which constitutes just a leather strap and buckle, can have so many subtleties, but like your shoes it says a great deal about your taste level.

Spend as much money as you can on a belt but don't show the wealth with monograms or prominent lettering. Quality leather will last and look better for longer and also remember that the belt has a job to do. Long gone are the days of a prominent "look at my groin" shiny buckle. The belt has become anonymous and should be barely seen, as such it has become thinner and more matt or aged-looking. Here are some tips on choosing one.

★ Colourwise, stick to black or brown leather and don't worry too much about it matching your shoes.

★ Don't fasten it too tight as this will ruch up your waistband and make you look as if your trousers don't fit; if too loose, the belt will shift around.

★ Crocodile or alligator skins can leave you looking a little like an African despot if they are too showy, so keep the wealth on the downlow.

★ In the summer months you can have fun with coloured fabric belts, which look great with shorts, but make sure the belt is the correct length. Never allow the excess to hang down as though you're trying to say something about your manhood. It looks bad and, worst of all, cheap.

Braces

For an authentic look, you need to have the buttons in your trousers to accommodate braces (or "suspenders" as the Americans call them). The clip-on ones look a little "boy band" and flimsy. Choose braces with nice leather detailing and the security of decent support. They look cool on denim jeans and vintage-style under tweed suits. The thickness of the braces should be judged in proportion to you; the bigger you are, the thicker they should be.

Cufflinks

Keith Penton, department head of jewellery at Christie's auction house in London, explains here the history of the cufflink and why, together with the signet ring and watch, it is one of the few pieces of jewellery acceptable for men to wear.

"Whether classical or avant-garde, set with precious metal or plastic, cufflinks provide the perfect opportunity for a man to wear his art on his sleeve. Cufflinks, as we know them, first appeared in the late eighteenth century and evolved from sleeve buttons.

"Previously the wristbands of a shirt had small openings either side through which a thin ribbon or string was passed to hold the sleeve closed. Surviving pairs of early sleeve links are often set with colourless paste (a lead-based glass), coloured agates, and sometimes rock crystal with compartments for hair or miniature portraits and are frequently mounted in silver with pieced bar or figure-of-eight connecting links between the two plaques or buttons.

For centuries men had worn a profusion of jewels of different types, but gradually this declined until the early nineteenth century when Benjamin Disraeli excited comment for wearing a variety of studs, rings, chains, fob seals and stickpins. By the early 1900s a signet ring and a pair of cufflinks were the only acceptable jewellery for a gentleman. Hardly surprising then, with so few opportunities for display, that cufflinks have retained their appeal and become ever more collectable. The fact that they still perform a function is also in their favour. Designs range from bars, hoops, spheres, knots, animals, to every shape of plaque that you can dream of, some with chain connections, others with bars of different types, folding terminals and patented mechanisms. Some connoisseurs only accept double-sided plaques; others are happy to have a single decorative link with a swivelling post and bar fitting, which they maintain is easier to use.

"The gift of cufflinks is something of a rite of passage and complete dress sets, including links, waistcoat buttons and shirt studs for use with white tie, are still sought-after for eighteenth and twenty-first birthday presents. These often have fitted cases, and even though the opportunity for formal dress is much more limited nowadays, the giving of a dress set is somewhat symbolic. Typically they range from hexagonal to circular panels and are usually made from white gold or platinum inset with onyx, rock crystal or mother-of-pearl with a central diamond or seed pearl accent."

Period Cufflinks

Keith Penton gives further advice on period cufflinks here and in the tips below. "Late Victorian and Edwardian gold cufflinks can range from the relatively plain to an enamelled pair depicting game birds or another sporting subject, or the four vices (usually depicting playing cards, a bottle of champagne, a horse and jockey, and a dancing girl!).

"Another popular type were set with rock crystal cabochons, carved from the reverse and painted with dogs, animals and sporting themes. Known variously as reverse intaglio or Essex crystals, the appearance from the front gives a three-dimensional effect. Cheaper costume copies were prevalent in the 1930s using moulded glass, but these are quite crude in comparison.

"The crème de la crème of cufflinks were produced in the early twentieth century by the great jewellery houses from Cartier to Van Cleef & Arpels, Boucheron and Fabergé, to name but a few. They range from delicately engraved and enamelled examples featuring pastel-coloured enamel and rose-cut diamonds to bolder geometric patterns and the strong chromatic contrasts of the Art Deco period. Some of the most popular designs are still in production today, including the Cartier stirrup cufflink with folding ring terminals and the reeded batons of Van Cleef & Arpels with a plain or gem-set central band (the baton slides through the central hoop and ingeniously clicks into place) and can command high prices at auction.

"Throughout the 1960s and '70s cufflink designs were often quite sculptural with textured nuggets, abstract shapes and random scatterings of gem stones reflecting the gold work of the period – this style is now much more appreciated after languishing throughout the 1980s and '90s."

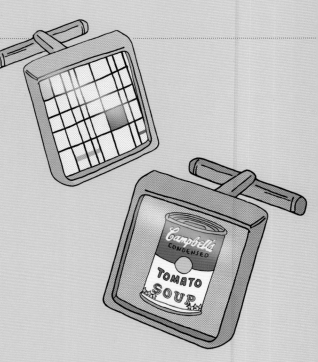

Buying Antique Cufflinks

★ If contemplating a pair of double-sided cufflinks with chain connections, check that the panel of the cufflink will fit through your buttonhole. Also bear in mind that a small panel may fall through a soft cuff and come undone too readily (shirts were starched in the nineteenth century and provided more resistance).

★ Beware that very bulky cufflinks might be uncomfortable to wear if working at a desk or keyboard.

★ Cufflinks that have been in regular use for 80 years may have very worn chain links/connections and these might be expensive to repair.

★ Check vintage enamel cufflinks as they are often chipped and may have had later restoration. The price or auction estimate should reflect this.

★ Check that the links are a true pair – a single double-side link is often divided and bar backs added to form a working set. Also, after a loss replacement copies are sometimes commissioned, so look out for subtle differences and changes in the colour of the gold. Waistcoat buttons are often converted to links with the addition of a detachable S-shaped link, which is not really a problem if the plaques all match.

★ Study genuine Edwardian enamel cufflinks and be aware that there are later copies available.

★ Buy from a reputable source and ask a specialist for their opinion.

Watches

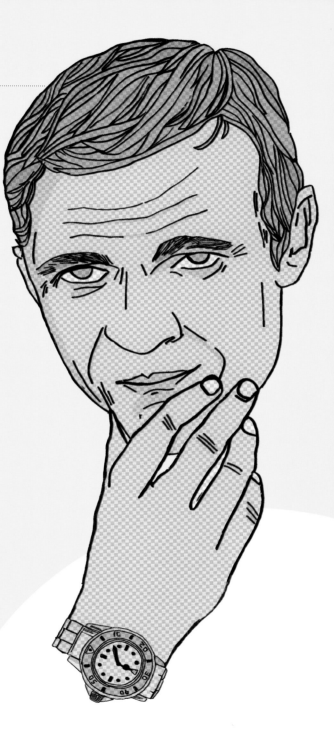

A watch is a man's most important item of jewellery. Most men would be lost without theirs, however they can go into the stratosphere of pricing. There is always a better, more expensive, razzle-dazzle timepiece around the corner and, to be totally honest, some of the really expensive ones are just as ugly as the cheaper ones. This is going to sound ignorant about the inner workings but generally, for The Chic Geek, it's the outside that counts. A respected name is fantastic and fills you with confidence but for purely visual purposes, a watch should be judged on its proportions and design.

★ Choose a watch that is in proportion to your wrist. If you have small wrists don't be afraid to purchase a women's style, which is often a better sizing.

★ Diamonds and blinging elements should definitely be left to the girls. Yellow gold watches are also a big no-no unless you happen to sell used cars.

★ Some watches are investments and as such they will last a lifetime; others are fun and colourful. Always have a fun watch for the summer as nobody wants to take their Patek Philippe to the beach.

★ A stainless-steel bracelet is great for everyday use and a leather or exotic skin strap is perfect for the evening but make sure it fits the wrist. There is nothing worse than a baggy watch sliding up and down somebody's wrist.

★ An expensive watch is more likely to be scratch- and water-resistant and will look better over time but each watch has its own merits so look at the description before you purchase. If you have any questions or are spending a lot of money, go to an established jeweller.

★ Collecting watches can quickly become addictive. A decent watch will always be worth something.

★ Avoid fashion watches because you're just paying for the name. Choose somebody who is a master in their craft, whether be it Swatch or Jaeger-LeCoultre.

Hats

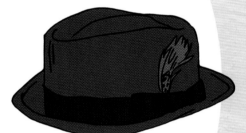

There is the practical hat and then there is the statement hat. The first is a beanie or a trapper hat in winter to keep your head warm or a straw hat in summer to shade your head; the latter is really dodgy ground for a man.

Apart from when worn as uniform or the afore-mentioned practicalities, most hats get hijacked by the "look-at-me" brigade. Hat-wearing is an art and, as such, it takes a knack to pull it off. The male hat should be subtle and part of the overall outfit; it should not be an attention-seeking beacon on your head. There are as many types of hat as there are people and here are thoughts on a few.

Baseball Cap So common as to become invisible, this makes a good choice for anyone who wishes to remain anonymous.

Beanie The winter hat of choice for the young man with one downside – difficult to take off without exposing a suffocated hairstyle.

Boater Very English public schoolboy but gaining ground in an eccentric summery way.

Bowler You'll probably never wear one of these, unless you're going as a *Clockwork Orange* droog for fancy dress.

Bucket or rain hat This is the type babies wear in the sun and can look really cute, especially as a waterproof hat.

Flat cap Alright, Guv'nor? A bit traditional London East End gangster or Joe Pesci in *Goodfellas*. A traditional tweed cap, when the right proportion to your head, looks cool. Stick to classic colours and fabrics.

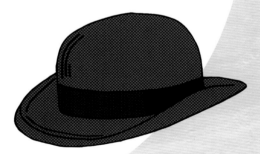

Panama Traditional in a pompous, middle-England type of way, but when worn right can be quite rakish.

Trapper A sheepskin or fur trapper perfectly covers the ears and keeps your head warm; also looks good with classic American workwear. Choose a fur that has been shaved or is short, otherwise the hat can look too large.

Trilby A little large for today's tastes.

Top hat For a day at the horse races and weddings only. A beautiful hat, especially when made of silk.

Manbags

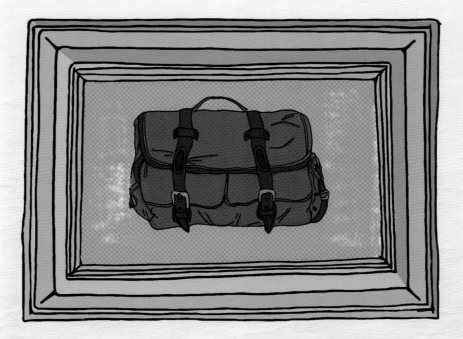

The moniker "manbag" has become something of a derogatory term for any type of bag a man carries. It has often been regarded as a feminine trait for a man to have a bag but sometimes our pockets aren't enough. Men have taken to bags like ducks to water and all shapes and styles have become increasingly present in the male wardrobe. You don't have to stick to one shape all the time – you can mix it up a bit.

When choosing a bag, it is all about proportions; too small it looks feminine, too large and it's impractical and heavy to carry. With leather goods, generally the more money you spend, the better the quality. Invest in a good-quality bag as they can take some serious battering and need to handle the everyday strain. Here are some thoughts on current styles.

Attaché/Briefcase The briefcase, if in a small format, can be très chic. Go for something well-crafted and sturdy.

Duffel/Gym bag Although this type can be a bit bulbous, the small nylon papillon-shaped gym bag has gained popularity among the retro crowd.

Messenger This usually sits on a large strap across the body. The downside is that this can disrupt the line of your outfit, plus you have to pull it off over your head.

Portfolio Case A bit like a male version of the clutch. Quite impractical but can look good if held at arm's length.

Rucksack Strictly for casual wear, this type is comfortable to wear but can look a bit young and touristy.

Shopper Like a tote but made from fabric or light-weight material, this looks good and does your bit for the environment at the checkout counter.

Tote This has become the fashionable smart bag. Held at arm's length, never on the crook of the arm, the tote is very chic.

Washbag Style Leave this one to the footballers. It's far too feminine and you have to hold it like petting a small dog.

Shoes

Shoes are the full stop to any outfit: people look at you, then scan down and make an assessment of your taste levels by looking at your feet. Don't let them down! You can get away with a lot if you've got good shoes.

A good shoe is all about proportions; you don't want your feet to look like canoes. Certain styles and shapes will make your feet look smaller or bigger and suit certain sizes of feet more than others. A man's shoe should make his feet look elegant, not clumpy or bigger than they actually are, but still retain an air of masculinity. Always keep your shoes in good order and clean. Distressed or aged is fine; shabby chic is cool.

Smart Shoes

Brogue The are lots of different types of brogue to choose from. Look for ones with very defined detailing, as this is a sign of quality.

Chelsea Boot Very swinging '60s, the Chelsea boot looks good with a bit of heel and when slim to the foot. Wear with slim/tapered trousers.

Lace-up Oxford This is your classic everyday smart shoe. There are lots of variations, but the classic is still a solid black round toe.

Loafer The loafer is a slip-on shoe that comes in lots of different styles, from the penny to tassel to the snaffle. Look for one that tapers at the end and has quality detailing such as multi-tassels or a metal snaffle. This shoe looks good with slim/tapered trousers, showing a bit of sock.

Monk Strap This has become quite an interesting and formal shoe. The double straps on the side show an old-school refinement. This shoe is something different yet traditional to try.

Patent This shiny dress shoe is traditionally worn with dinner suits, but now comes in a multitude of colours. A patent shoe can add a touch of sleekness to an outfit, but still stick to after-dark to wear them.

Slipper Not the type to keep your feet warm! This is the king-of-the-castle, look-at-me, embroidered number in coloured velvet. Wear these instead of patent as a dress shoe and look for different designs: skulls, initials, crowns or go plain. The best slippers have satin quilting inside and a heel.

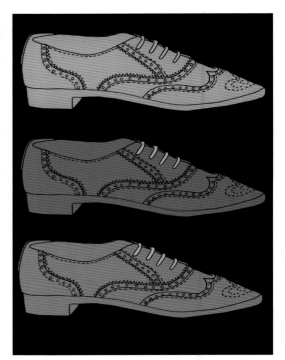

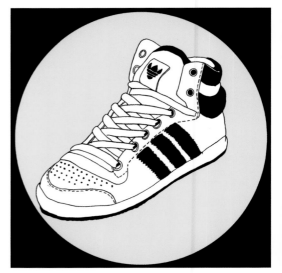

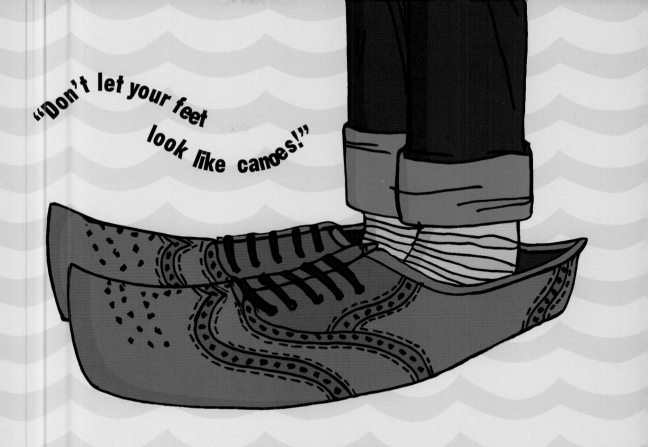

"Don't let your feet look like canoes!"

Casual Shoes

Desert Boot Every man should own a pair of desert boots, which will take you anywhere. A very democratic shoe, it can say anything you want about you. A year-round favourite is brown suede.

Dr Martens DMs or a multi-eyelet high boot is the traditional style of boot. These forever come in and out of style, from the army to skinheads to robust winter footwear, and are as tough as old boots.

Trainers The trainer (sneaker) is a whole different look and the advice for these is to leave the technical stuff to the sports field. Buy something comfortable and minimal in terms of design and colour.

Seasonal Shoes

Boat Shoe Deck shoes, topsiders, call them what you will, the boat shoe is the smart summer shoe. Look for the different detailing with the laces and a variety of colour combinations. Wear sans socks.

Espadrilles These are a cheap and simple summer shoe that has a plain cotton top with a jute rope sole. Wear them like outdoor slippers.

Flip-flops These should definitely not be worn away from water.

Sandal The sandal has come on in leaps and bounds in the men's fashion department. Taking the lead from women's designs, we now have everything from gladiators to Birkenstocks. Choose styles that have a lightness about them and also in a colour that complements your skin tone. Toes become important with sandals, so keep this in mind and don't be afraid to give your toenails some TLC pre-sandal season.

Formal Dress

There will be moments in your life when you'll be asked to dress up and they'll be other times when you'll want to do so. Formalwear doesn't have to be old-fashioned, staid or fussy; you can still stamp your personality on this smart "uniform".

The traditional black-tie dinner jacket (tuxedo) is usually a single-breasted jacket in a black mohair/wool mix with matching trousers that have a silk "tuxedo" stripe down the leg. These suits can appear quite boxy so opt for elegance and go for a one-button version with a shawl collar.

Patterned evening jackets are becoming quite the thing. Still meant to be worn with plain black trousers, they add a dash of retro playboy to your look. The idea of evening clothes is to wear something that suits a candle-lit environment, so think rich velvets, sumptuous silks and patent leather. Accessories like velvet bow-ties and silk pocket squares will help with this effect. Just because an invite says "black tie" doesn't mean you can't play around with patterns and colour so long as the items suit the evening theme.

Formal Accessories

★ Patent shoes are a good choice; the slip-on ones with silk bows have just the right amount of irony for any stylish man.

★ Cummerbunds are too much nowadays and fussy. Avoid packs of bow-tie and matching cummerbunds at all costs.

★ Unless it's a formal business event, have fun with evening clothes. Thickly rimmed spectacles or a flash of colourful cashmere sock add cheeky panache to your James Bond evening persona.

★ If you really want to stand out or feel brave, try bold tartan trousers with a velvet shawl-collar jacket and matching bow-tie for a Scottish evening style.

Wearing Morning Dress

Holland & Sherry, suppliers of the finest Yorkshire and Scottish cloth to prestigious tailors and luxury brands, here give advice on how to wear morning dress. In 1836 Stephen George Holland and Frederick Sherry began the business as woollen merchants at 10 Old Bond Street, London, specializing in both woollen and silk cloths. By 1900 the firm was exporting to many countries and around that time a sales office was established in New York. In the early part of the twentieth century, the United Kingdom, Europe, North and South America were the dominant markets for the company. By 1982 the business moved to Savile Row, which remains the registered head office.

The name "morning dress" originates from the nineteenth-century practice of wearing a cutaway-front single-breasted coat for riding a horse in the morning. Hence the American term "cutaway", meaning a morning coat. A common mistake is to call morning dress a tuxedo. It is incorrect to wear morning dress to any formal or informal evening event, but for events taking place before 5 pm, such as weddings, funerals, state functions and Royal Ascot for example, morning dress can be worn. The morning dress elements consist of:

★ Morning coat in black or grey worsted wool.

★ Waistcoat in black or light grey worsted, either single- or double-breasted.

★ Trousers in grey striped worsted wool with a single pleat and no turn-up (trouser cuff). Supported by braces (suspenders).

★ Shirt in white cotton or linen with a double cuff.

★ Tie or cravat in any colour of silk.

★ Black Oxford shoes with a plain toecap (not patent leather).

★ Top hat in black or grey silk (optional).

★ Gloves in suede, chamois or kid leather (optional).

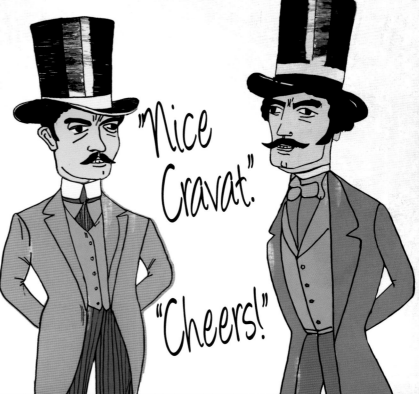

"Nice Cravat."

"Cheers!"

Casual Dressing

Everyday or casual dressing is where you need to perfect your confidence. What a man looks like on his dress down is the tell-tale of his innermost style. If you can get your mufti dress looking good then everything else will slide into place. Use a capsule wardrobe (see page 77) as your base, then work the details or nuances of your daily dressing to give you individual flair. Your everyday look shouldn't be laboured over but instead appear as if it comes naturally. Details usually come in the form of accessories, items such as watches, scarves, shoes and socks.

A man shouldn't be decorated like a Christmas tree and less is most definitely more. Become your own editor and pick a small selection of things you like and they will naturally work together. Don't be afraid of colour; think of it as a highlight, a full stop or an underline of you.

Often it's not what you wear but how you wear it. Everyday dressing requires an element of imagination. You shouldn't just take what you are given by the manufacturer or designer and wear it that way; play around until it suits you better or reflects the weather or where you are going.

This is where you are introduced to the fashion verb "tszuj", pronounced "zhuj". In fashion circles this is the word which best describes the tweaking of your outfit and separates a stylish man from a layman. "Tszujing" is the simple matter of rolling up the sleeves on a shirt or pushing up the arms on a jacket, or the size of the turn-ups on your jeans. Changing these areas or details tightens and fine-tunes your look. Play around and see what works for you. Like a fashion Rubik's Cube, you change one thing and this can alter something else, so continue tweaking until you feel happy.

It's all about fit, fit, fit. Don't worry about labels or digits; take a few sizes of the same item into the changing room and try them all on and see what works. Different shapes work better or worse in different sizes so don't get hung up on your sizing; the mirror will tell you which size you are. Remember fitted, but not too tight.

Try to be appropriate and practical, dress for your destination and appropriately for the weather. The weather will dictate a lot, but you work with this, not against it. Also, there are different ways to do the same thing; for example if you're cold in the summer, choose something warm yet seasonal such as a linen sweater or more layers, rather than a winter bodywarmer.

NEVER EVER FASHIONS

There is a time and a place for everything and judging that is something you will learn but The Chic Geek does have a small list of
NEVER EVERS:

Leather trousers

Medallions

Monogrammed luggage

Thongs

Mankinis

Mullets

Acid-wash denim

Sovereign rings

Bandanas

Fake fur

Cuban heels

Goatees

Cubic Zirconia

Penazzle

Merkin

Shopping Guide

Shopping is an art form and like most art forms there are amateurs and professionals. The difference is intelligent consumerism; knowing exactly where to get what you want and what you are paying for. The clever shopper knows the difference between value and price: price is an indicator of an item but not the "be all and end all". A discerning male buyer can spot quality from just from a piece of fabric sticking out of a rail. The label is also a guideline but it's a mixture of design, quality, price and that certain *je ne sais quoi* which makes an item worth buying.

★ Know what you already have and where the gaps are.

★ Focus. Walking around aimlessly or searching the internet can leave you feeling overwhelmed and bored.

★ Always buy the best of its type. If you don't find it, wait.

★ Nobody has a limitless budget. Break it down and allocate larger funds for coats and leather goods.

★ Labels are signs to be read. A designer name doesn't necessarily mean the best quality. Look at the labels inside the garments, see where things are made and what material they are constructed from. This will tell you a lot about the item.

★ Don't be afraid to ask why something is the price it is. The store will probably give you more background and justification. For example, you can tell real crocodile by the line of zeros on the end of the price!

★ Look at the model images and mannequins in the shop. They are there for inspiration and to give you ideas on how to wear things.

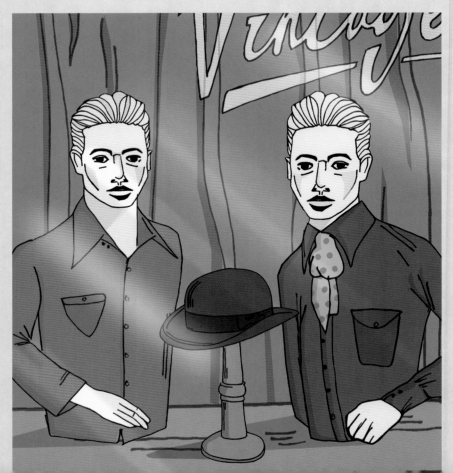

How to Shop the Sales

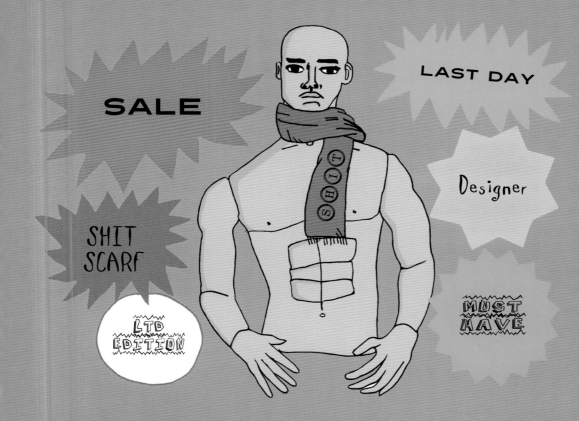

We all love a bargain, but sometimes our judgement can be clouded by the discounts. Here's a guide to staying focused during sale season.

① Don't be seduced by the label; designers make mistakes.

② Make sure the item fits really well. You really want it, we understand that, but if it doesn't fit, it won't look any good and you should walk away.

③ It might be on the sale rail for a reason. Think before you buy, and inspect the item for flaws.

④ Buy classics. Spend the same money that you would pre-sale but buy better quality – white shirts, blue jeans, grey and navy V-necks, black shoes, leather belts.

⑤ Stock up on quality staples. Save money by buying your favourite underwear, socks, T-shirts, knitwear, night clothes and accessories at discounted prices.

⑥ Have a look on the first and last day. If you like something, particularly online, watch it and swoop as soon as the price is right.

Vintage Shopping

Because vintage is such a vast and subjective subject, nothing you do can be an exact science. Spending hours on eBay, or days looking in musty-smelling vintage shops, can have you feeling down-hearted and empty-handed or euphoric from striking vintage gold. There is nothing quite like the feeling of finding something special that fits and is affordable. Remember, though, beauty is in the eye of the beholder, there is an art to nailing down the best pieces at reasonable prices.

1 The strongest advice is to be informed. Obvious I know, but soak up information like a sponge. Be knowledgeable about fashion history, motifs and labels, decide what you like and then look for the best places to find it. You will learn as you go, discovering new labels and brands, which is part of the fun. One often leads to another.

2 True vintage isn't about saving money, and it's not about dressing cheaply. It's about appreciating a particular piece or era. The amount you spend on vintage can range from a few pounds to thousands of pounds. However much you spend, it's about looking individual and playing with history and styles.

3 Price is dependent on a variety of factors: the condition, the label/designer or era and the quality of the garment – which is usually deciphered by the name on the label, rarity or whether the item is in "fashion" and therefore in demand. The best things were usually expensive when new, so don't expect to pick them up for nothing. People are very clued up today, but we can always hope for something that slips through the net!

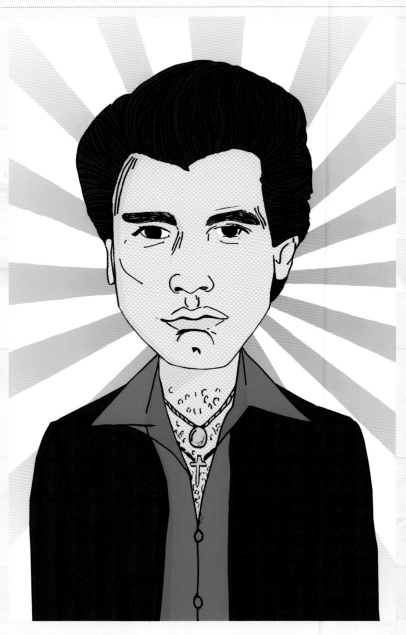

4 Train your eye. You'll see rail upon rail of clothes in certain places and you'll need to be able to spot something of quality and style among all the less interesting stuff. The places you have to rummage usually sell cheaper items, so having a good eye will save you money and also time. You can often spot a gem from an interesting colour or piece of material sticking out.

5 Fit is very important. If you can't wear it, or it is ill-fitting, then what is the point? It does help to be a bit slimmer in this game as our fore-fathers were generally smaller both in terms of height and girth. Tailored items can be difficult to find without alteration and if altering, factor this into the price when buying something and make sure you will be able to find somebody experienced enough to carry out the work.

6 Keep your eye on trends and current fashions as this will give you an idea on how to integrate vintage into your wardrobe. It will also make the item contemporary. You will see "vintage inspired" items being re-made and as we all know, nothing beats an original.

7 One of the attractions of vintage is the idea of wearing history; that authentic feeling you get. Yet vintage fashion shouldn't look like costume and wearing vintage should be a non-obvious form of dressing. The art of mixing vintage is to choose pieces that feel contemporary or sit well in contemporary fashion.

8 An emotional connection is the deal sealer; picture yourself wearing it. Think about what else you own that will go with it and where and when you'll be able to wear it. Some things you just can't put down.

9 Buy the best you can afford. In terms of investment, they will hold their value more, or maybe increase in value if you've bought well.

10 Don't forget to enjoy the item. Vintage fashion should be enjoyed; if something is too precious, you will have to decide whether you want to risk wearing it or not.

11 Haggle. Dealers expect to negotiate on the price.

12 Beware of fakes. This especially applies to designer leather goods, Louis Vuitton trunks and the like, which are definitely items not to buy online. If you're unsure, always buy from a reputable dealer or antiques market that has been authenticated. And if the price is too good to be true, then it probably is. Be very wary.

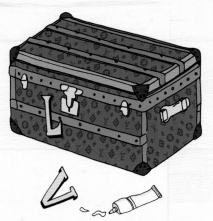

13 Have the element of fantasy. Vintage allows you be indulgent and experimental without the price. You may buy things you only wear once a year, such as smoking jackets or plus fours, but they are nice to have. Wardrobes should be regarded as a collection that you add to.

14 Build a relationship with the dealer of your favourite store. Consult and use their knowledge. Most of the best stuff never makes it into the shop since the dealer has buyers waiting for things. By letting them know what you're looking for, hopefully you'll get first dibs of anything that may be of interest to you.

15 When buying something expensive it is best to see it in the flesh first. Use the Internet to search for things, but if you're making a big purchase it is always best to check it out.

16 Charity shops are still worth a rummage but the reason you go to vintage stores is because they have done a lot of the time-consuming research for you, hence the reason you pay a premium. Usually the more edited the shop, the more expensive the items, but they do save you time.

17 Study the details. The buttons, fabric, pattern, cut – these are what make something special. They will also signal if a piece is of quality.

18 Like the rest of fashion, some vintage items will come in and out of style. Something that looked good before may no longer seem "cool". If something is special, hold on to it; if not, then see if you can get anything for it from a dealer or vintage shop.

The Holy Grail of Men's Vintage

There are certain items that run through the history of men's fashion which don't diminish in desirability over time. They are proudly labelled with the adjective "timeless'" and are the status symbols of any stylish man. These items transcend the normal rules of fashion and have earned their place in the vintage hall of fame. Men's vintage collectors would sell their grandmother to own a few of these items. Welcome to the Holy Grail of Men's Vintage.

Gucci Loafers Nothing says "timeless" like a Gucci loafer. It was in 1966 that Gucci took the further step of adding the horse bit metal detailing on the front. It has become an icon of twentieth-century style. They still do many variations today but the best era for Gucci was the jet-setting 1970s.

Hermès H Belt Synonymous with the Sloane Ranger, the Hermès H belt is pure status symbol. Its full name is the Constance H belt and it was first produced in the 1950s. Incredibly expensive for a simple leather strap and metal H on the front, it says "money".

Burberry Trenchcoat The most famous of its type, the first Burberry trench was submitted by Thomas Burberry, the inventor of gabardine fabric, as a design for an army officer's raincoat to the UK's War Office in 1901. It became an optional item of dress in the British Army and was obtained by private purchase by officers and Warrant Officers Class I who were under no obligation to own them. No other ranks were permitted to wear them. It has now become another twentieth-century icon and, thanks to creative director Christopher Bailey, a twenty-first century classic.

Mid-century Cowboy Shirt The cowboy shirt is one of the most masculine items of any man's wardrobe. It conjures up a testosterone-fuelled image of horseriding cowboys in the prairies of the American Midwest. The cowboy shirt has had many reincarnations and in 1946, Jack A Weil, better known as Jack A, invented the first snap-buttoned cowboy shirt. The shirts from this era and the 1950s are the most collectable.

Classic Pucci Emilio Pucci started designing in the late 1940s and is typically known for his womenswear. His highly patterned, bright silks have become its trademark and a timeless dose of Capri sunshine. For men, look for Pucci ties and the odd shirt. Pricey.

Louis Vuitton Trunk The Louis Vuitton label was founded by Monsieur Vuitton in 1854 on rue Neuve des Capucines in Paris. In 1858, Monsieur Vuitton introduced his flat-bottom trunks with trianon canvas, making them lightweight and airtight. Before the introduction of Vuitton's trunks, rounded-top trunks were used, generally to promote water run-off, and thus could not be stacked. It was Vuitton's grey Trianon canvas flat trunk that became famous for stacking for ease with voyages. Becoming successful and prestigious, many other luggage makers began to imitate LV's style and design. Along with the other French luggage label Goyard, they are the ultimate in luxury trunks. Expect to pay a lot for one of these babies.

Missoni from the 1970s Ottavio and Rosita Missoni married in April 1953 and set up a small knitwear workshop in Gallarate, not far from Rosita's home village in Italy. In 1958 they presented their first collection in Milan called Milano-Simpathy, which was the first to bear the Missoni label. They are famous for their highly colourful, striped knitwear, which has become their signature. The best vintage pieces are from the 1970s.

Leather Gladstone Bag The classic Victorian bag, the Gladstone is also known as a doctor's bag. Named after the four-times prime minister, William Ewart Gladstone, the bag is a small portmanteau suitcase built over a rigid frame that could separate into two equal sections. Renowned for the amount of travelling he did, the Gladstone is typically made of stiff leather and often belted with lanyards. You can often pick them up in junk shops, but those in prime condition and by a good maker fetch big money.

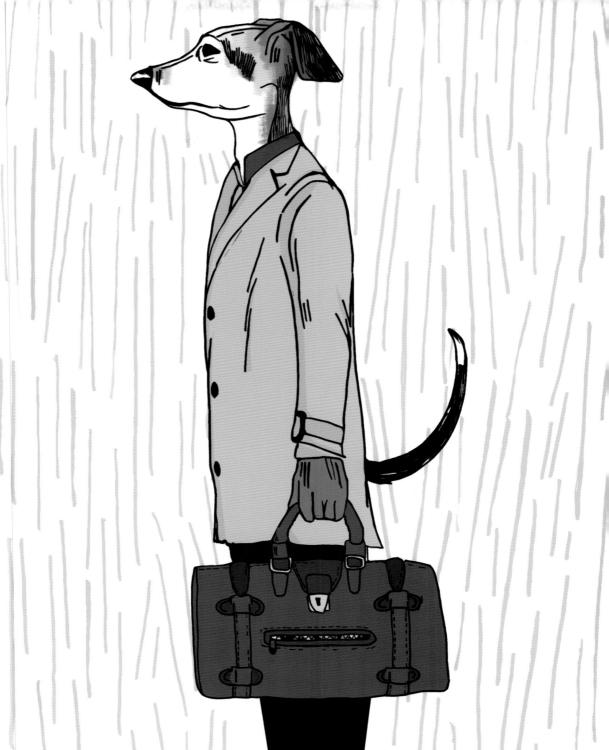

Something "Of Its Era"

This should be the fun part of vintage – the section of vintage that screams of its era but can be easily mixed up to be modern.

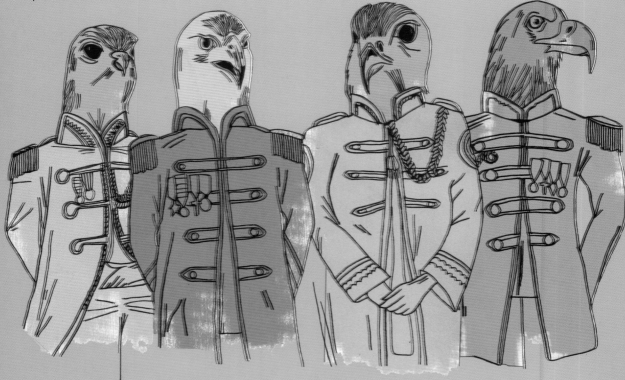

Leather Jacket A leather jacket is a prime example, especially if it has that 1970s, Elton John-style arrows on the collar or it is made by Zilli, the Lyon-based French luxury men's label. Look for fine quality with great detailing.

Military Jacket From the Beatles to the Libertines, the military jacket has been a cliché, yet something inside of you still wants one. They first came into style during the 1960s, thanks to forward-looking shops such as "I Was Lord Kitchener's Valet". This Portobello Road clothing boutique achieved a period of fame in 1960s Swinging London by promoting antique military uniforms as fashion items. Peter Blake the artist who designed the Beatles' *Sgt. Pepper's Lonely Hearts Club Band* album cover said that he and Paul McCartney got the idea for the album sleeve when they were walking together past the "I Was Lord Kitchener's Valet" shop.

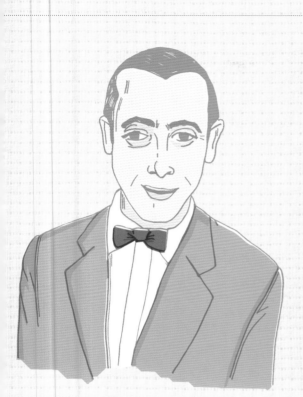

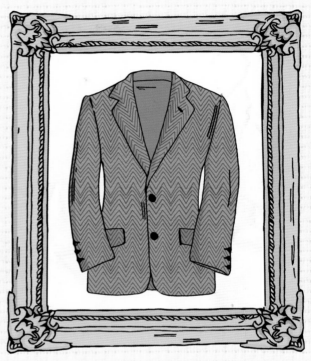

1950s Clip-On American Bow-ties The bow-tie returned a few years back with a strong dose of irony. These skinny, clip-on American bow-ties sum up the 1950s, a time of burger joints and drive-thrus. Relatively cheap and a nice thing to collect, brands to look for include Ormond NYC or Wembley.

Harris Tweed This is the ultimate in tweed. Harris Tweed is the only fabric protected by an act of parliament. If it hasn't got the orb motif then it isn't Harris tweed. Hand-woven by islanders on the Isles of Harris, Lewis, Uist and Barra in the Outer Hebrides of Scotland using local wool, every length of cloth produced is stamped with the official Orb symbol, trademarked by the Harris Tweed Association in 1909 when Harris Tweed was defined as "hand-spun, hand-woven and dyed by the crofters and cottars in the Outer Hebrides". The Harris Tweed Authority took over from the Harris Tweed Association in 1993 by Act of Parliament. Thus the definition of Harris Tweed became statutory and forever tied the cloth to the Islands: "Harris Tweed means a tweed which has been hand-woven by the islanders at their homes in the Outer Hebrides, finished in the islands of Harris, Lewis, North Uist, Benbecula, South Uist and Barra and their several purtenances (the Outer Hebrides) and made from pure virgin wool dyed and spun in the Outer Hebrides."

Future Vintage

It's not easy finding good men's vintage. Unlike women, men had smaller wardrobes and also wore their clothes out, therefore there isn't much left! So here The Chic Geek has looked into the metro-sexual wardrobes of the last 10 to 15 years and decide what is worth keeping and what will, one day, maybe, become vintage. When something is good, be it in quality or design, it will always be desirable. Here are his tips for future men's vintage.

Anything Tailored by Alexander McQueen Even if McQueen hadn't passed away his pieces would still have been collectable. He came to prominence during the mid-1990s and anything bought in his first Conduit Street shop in London during this time is highly desirable. This is McQueen before he sold out to the Gucci Group. The menswear wasn't as provocative as the women's yet it was cut so well. McQueen took traditional British menswear but added his own strict and distinctive take.

Minimalism One of the defining trends of the 1990s, the purity of minimalist pieces often left people wondering what the fuss was all about. Designers such as Jil Sander, Helmut Lang and Prada all did a "less is more'" aesthetic during this time period.

Gucci "The Tom Ford Years" For most people, until Tom Ford arrived Gucci was a 1970s fashion label mentioned in a Sister Sledge song. The Texan injected his own egotistic sexiness that was so alluring that fashionistas just couldn't get enough. Gucci became one of the most desirable labels of the decade. The first collection, autumn/winter 1996, of blood-red velvet suits really cemented Tom Ford's look but it was the hippie collection of spring/summer 1999 that became iconic. The G men's thong and other publicity stunts made Tom Ford the master of self-promotion.

Miu Miu Menswear The final collection for this label was spring/summer 2008. Miu Miu, the younger brother of the Prada label, was less grown-up and serious. The only problem was availability. Some department stores and, for a short time, the small Miu Miu shop in London's Bond Street, sold the label but it was hard to get the show pieces. One notable collection was spring/summer 2002, which was a riot of Bermuda shorts printed with 1960s prints.

Christopher Bailey at Burberry In May 2001, Christopher Bailey arrived at Burberry and set about transforming the company into a very dynamic fashion house. His collections are always distinctive yet wearable and he makes Englishness international. Highlights during his years are his bright Pop Art collection in homage to David Hockney and the autumn/winter 2002 collection, which featured signature Burberry paisley.

Prada's Fun Accessories Italian label Prada has always produced cute little accessories such as teddybear-shaped key rings or robots to go with its collections, using a lot of these items to style the shows. A black gingerbread man from spring/summer 2003 was beautifully crafted in plastic and leather.

Dior Homme Hedi Slimane launched the Dior Homme label in 2000. He was previously head of menswear at YSL Rive Gauche, only leaving after the Gucci Group bought YSL and Tom Ford took over. With Dior Homme, Slimane defined and polished the super skinny male-size-zero, which resonated through the early years of the Noughties. The babyfood-eating designer took a strict approach with no compromise on the cut. The only problem was finding young manorexic men with the pockets deep enough to afford a Dior suit. The two didn't go together and in July 2007, Slimane decided to leave. His black skinny suit is probably the most collectable.

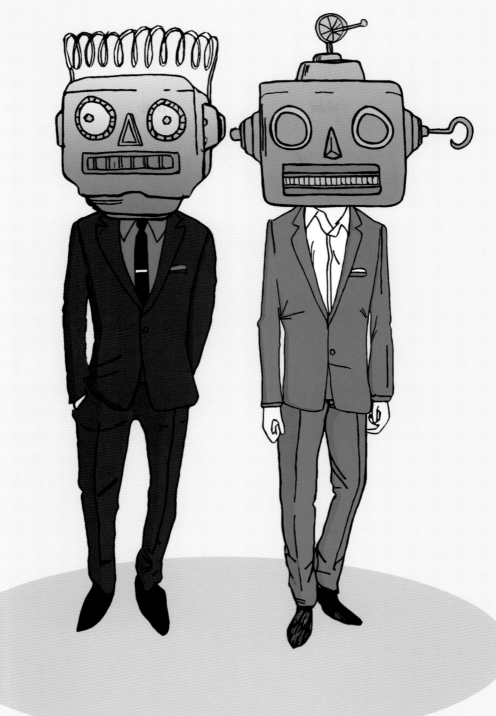

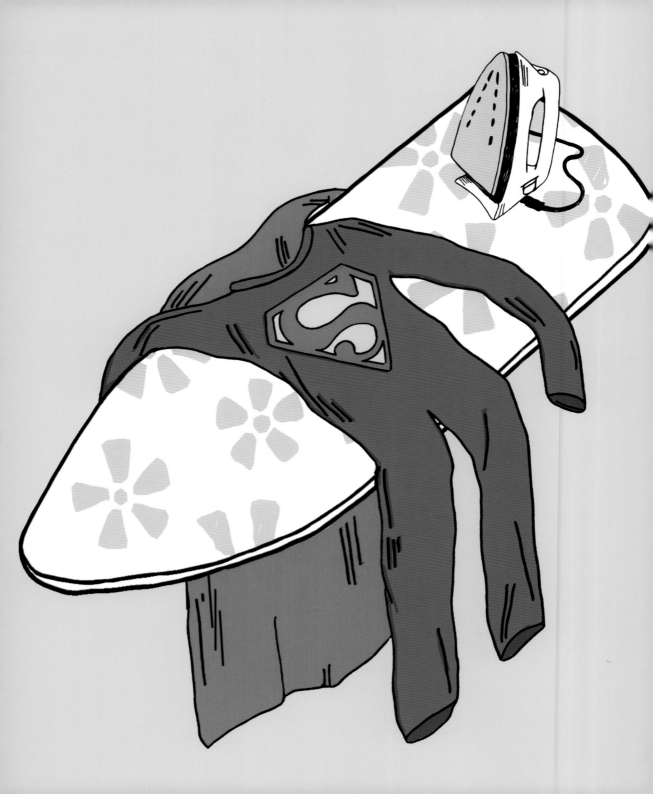

4 The Practical Geek

Time to get real. Looking good takes time, effort and know-how. You don't wake up one day knowing everything about getting dressed or looking after your clothes. This chapter is the engine room of your wardrobe, the place where you learn how to do the "boring" but necessary stuff.

A contemporary man stands on his own two feet and knows how to correctly wash his clothes or iron a shirt. The modern male is independent and can look after himself without an interfering Jeeves or shrinking his best Loro Piana sweater. You've spent all the time and expense finding and buying these lovely things, now you need to know how to look after them.

Following the guidelines over the next few pages will keep your garments looking their best and also make them last longer. Certain ways of doing things will save you time, be easier and give you a better result. We've asked a few experts in their fields for their personal advice plus The Chic Geek fills in the gaps on skills such as how to store your clothes, fold a shirt or shine your shoes. As we know, the devil is in the detail.

Now get to work!

How to Launder Your Clothes

Ideally, to keep our clothes looking their best we would never wash them, but hygienically, socially and psychologically this would never do. To look and feel our best, regular cleaning and washing of clothes is something unavoidable. Prevention is always better than cure, so be careful when you eat or drink, particularly around items that are difficult to clean or stain easily such as silk ties.

If you're wearing knitwear, wear something like an easy-to-wash T-shirt or vest between you and the knitwear. Tom Ford might famously go commando, but he has the budget! And it's always, always best to wear something between you and your trousers.

The smoking ban in most public buildings has helped to reduce the amount of dry-cleaning we need these days, particularly with coats and jackets, as that horrid, stale, post-party smoke smell is much less common. With coats and jackets, sponge any stains with water and see how they dry. If in doubt, ask your dry cleaner for advice with regard to a stain or fabric. Certain waterproofs, such as Mackintoshes and Barbours, cannot be dry-cleaned.

Machine Washing & Drying

★ Separate the colours and whites. Do this carefully so nothing crosses over and ruins the whites. Watch out for that pesky coloured sock that slips in!

★ Check the pockets. There is nothing worse than white tissue bits over everything or something important disappearing in the wash.

★ Close zippers as these can sometimes catch and damage other garments in the cycle.

★ Turn your jeans inside out before you wash them to preserve the colour better.

★ Pre-treat heavy stains with laundry detergent or stain remover, reading the instructions on the product label to check they're okay to use before you apply.

★ Always read the care labels on your garments. Don't be lazy and just shove everything in the machine. If you've invested time and money in buying something good, why ruin it by ignoring this last detail? If unsure, particularly with knitwear or fabric blends, hand-wash.

★ Wash towels separately so the lint doesn't go over everything else.

★ Use the measuring cap of the detergent bottle or the cup found in detergent boxes to measure out the exact amount of powder according to the manufacturer's instructions. If you are one of those men who buys the powder or detergent according to what's the best deal at the supermarket, read the application instructions because each brand and type will be different.

★ Check the dial at the front of the machine and set it according to your wash. There are different settings for different fabrics or load size.

★ Don't set the temperature too high; you may shrink the clothes, plus it is bad for the environment and it costs more money.

★ Hang out or dry your clothes straight away. There is nothing less attractive than that damp smell on clothing.

★ If you can, dry outside. Your clothes will smell better and it is kinder to the environment than using a dryer.

★ Always dry knitwear flat to stop it stretching and reshape when damp.

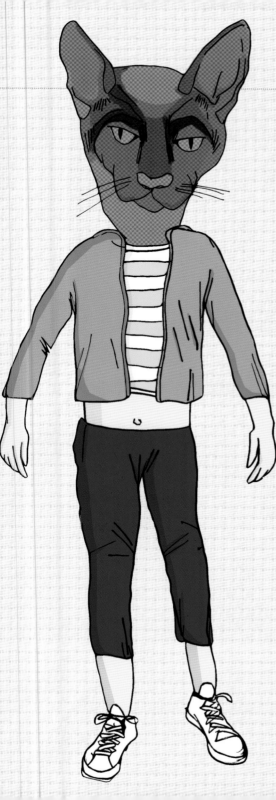

Hand Washing

If in doubt, hand-wash. It can be so disheartening to pull out a child-sized sweater from the washing machine and realize that it used to fit you. Your delicate clothes will last longer if they're not constantly subjected to the actions of the washing machine.

Buy some hand-washing detergent, read the label and add the recommended amount to the sink full of water. For the temperature of the water, look at the care instructions inside the garment.

Put your clothing in the water and get it thoroughly wet and soapy. If it's stained, you may want to let it soak for a while. Knead the clothing with your hands in the water for a few minutes. Unplug the sink, drain and start the water running. Rinse your clothing until the water runs clear, then rinse some more! Wring gently and hang to dry. Always dry knitwear flat to stop it stretching or losing its shape.

Removing Stains

First obvious note: be careful. Prevention is better than cure, so use your napkin or bring the plate up under your chin! But shit happens, so act quickly. If the garment can be easily removed without causing embarrassment, remove it and soak in cold water to loosen the stain. If the garment can't be removed, wet a cloth with cold water and blot until you've removed as much of the stain as possible. By rubbing it, you're only producing more damage to the fabric and may spread the stain. Once you're home, add a bit of washing-up liquid and continue to blot. You can pretreat with a laundry detergent or spot remover before using the washing machine. Never tumble dry or iron the stain as this will make it permanent. If the stain doesn't disappear, consult a dry-cleaner.

How to Iron a Shirt

Learning to iron a shirt properly is a rite of passage for any man. Practise makes perfect!

1 Choose a well-lit location with a clean area around it, as your shirt may touch the floor.

2 Make sure the ironing board is sturdy and the cover is clean and fits snugly onto the board.

3 Adjust the height of the ironing board so it is comfortable to iron and position the board the right way around, according to which hand you iron with.

4 Adjust the iron to the right temperature. If you are unsure what this should be, the care label on the shirt will say or the dial on the iron will indicate the different types of fabrics for heat settings.

5 Add water to the iron according to the manufacturer's instructions and turn the iron on to heat up.

6 If the shirt is very dry, dampen it first with a spray of water. Use the spray function on the iron or a spray bottle filled with water.

7 Place the shirt on the ironing board and then iron the collar from the points to the middle. Turn the shirt over and iron the back of the collar. This helps remove creases.

8 Next, take the shirt and pull it onto the tapered end of the ironing board so that the back of the yoke – the part of the shirt that sits on your shoulders – is flat on the board. Pull one shoulder into the tapered end of the ironing board and iron this half of the shoulder, then it over and do the same on the other side.

9 Sleeves can be a little harder to iron, so take your time and flatten out the fabric, avoiding big wrinkles before you apply the iron. First flatten one cuff on the ironing board and iron it. Then take that sleeve by the seam and lay the whole sleeve flat on the ironing board. If you can see the crease on the top of the sleeve from previous ironing, try to match it again so that you have a single crease line on the sleeve. Start at the top, where the sleeve is sewn onto the shirt, and work your way down to the cuff. Turn the sleeve over and iron the other side. Repeat with the other sleeve.

10 Now you're ready to iron the body of the shirt. With the collar to your left, place the left side of the shirt on the ironing board. On a man's shirt this is the side with the buttonholes. It may be easier to iron the upper portion by turning the shirt slightly so that the tapered part of the ironing board slips into the sleeve a little.

11 Iron around the collar carefully, as it is easy to cause a wrinkle here.

12 Next, pull the shirt flat on the ironing board again and iron the placket and the rest of the front left side.

13 Now rotate the shirt toward you so that half of the back is on the ironing board. Smooth it out with your hands and iron it. Keep rotating, smoothing, and ironing until you come to the right front of the shirt.

14 You can now put the shirt on a hanger. Check to see if there are any obvious wrinkles and give that area a quick spray with water and iron again.

15 Button the collar button and the next one or two buttons, which will help the shirt to keep its shape and button the collar buttons on Oxford shirts. Be careful not to crush the shirt when you put it in the wardrobe.

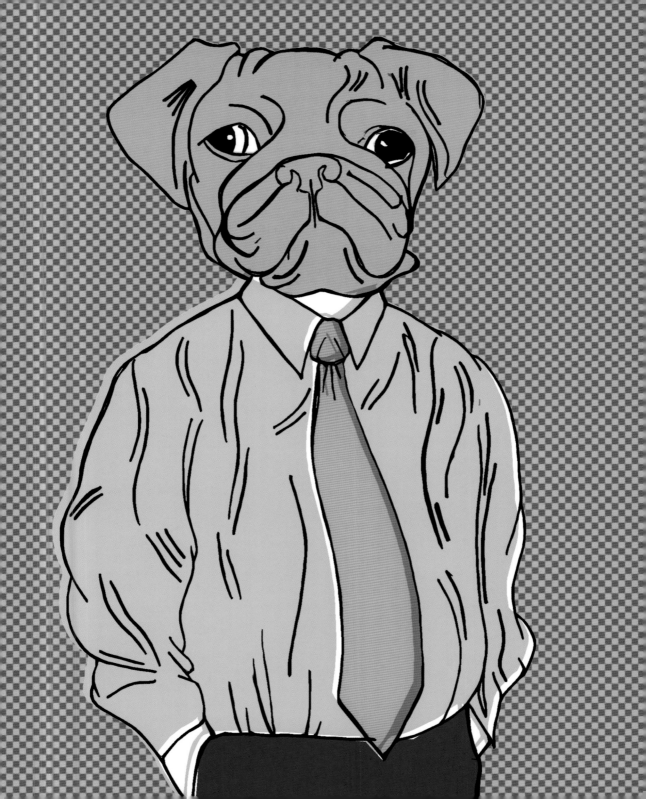

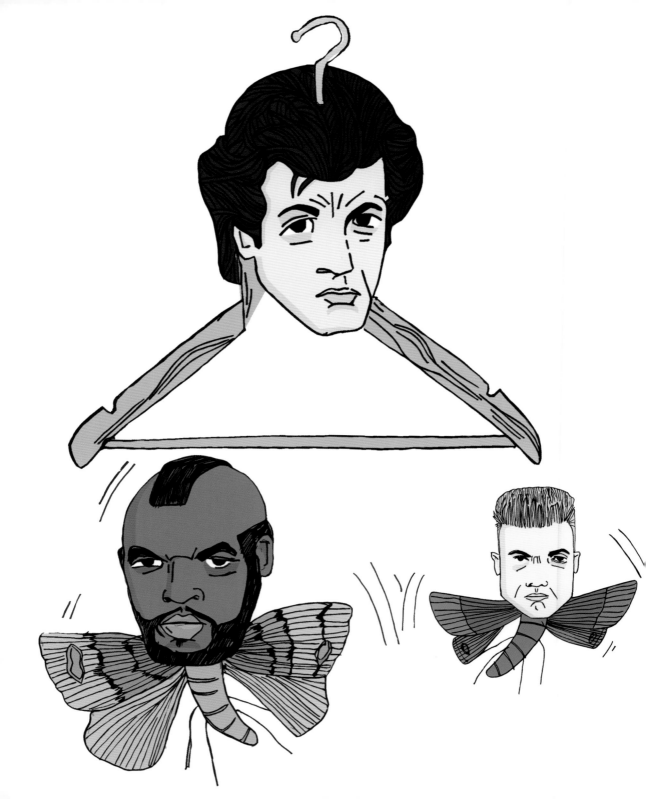

How to Store Your Clothes

The more we buy, the more we have to think about storage. Good storage will keep your clothes in perfect condition and also means you will be able to find everything quickly and you'll know exactly what you own. The Imelda Marcos' idea of storage isn't practical, so you need to be economical with space without crushing everything.

★ The places where you store your clothes should be cool, dry and dark. Sunlight, extreme heat and humidity can be damaging to clothing.

★ Clothing should have access to proper ventilation so as not to encourage mildew or mould.

★ Use wide hangers and not the wire ones from the dry cleaners, which will misshape your clothes.

★ Ideally, use hangers made from cedar wood, as this will repel moths.

★ Zip or button coats and jackets on the hangers to help them keep their shape.

★ With items you don't wear very often, use hanging garment bags but make sure they have some form of ventilation.

★ Keep drawers and wardrobes closed; also make sure boxes have lids to prevent dust or dirt getting in.

★ Watch out for moths or bugs. They and the larvae often live within the natural fibres of garments. If you find any, put the item in the freezer for 72 hours, which will kill larvae and eggs. When you have a major infestation, you may need to take more drastic action to eradicate them totally.

★ Make sure things are clean before you store them; insects are particularly attracted to the dirt.

★ Put shoetrees inside your shoes to help keep their shape.

How to Fold a Shirt

If you don't have the wardrobe space, you may want to fold your shirt. So, if you didn't spend your teenage years working at GAP, here's how.

① Button the top collar button, the third button and the bottom button.

② Lay the shirt face down on a flat surface, smoothing out any wrinkles.

③ Right side of the shirt first, fold about one-third of the body toward the centre of the shirt.

④ Fold the sleeve next. Create a fold at the shoulder. This should line up with the edge of the first body fold in the centre and the cuff should be sitting at the bottom end of the shirt. Make sure the sleeve keeps the crease in the arm.

⑤ Repeat for the other side.

⑥ Make a fold of several inches at the shirt-tail into the shirt, then fold again in half so the bottom edge is now under the collar.

⑦ Turn the shirt over, when it should look neat and square.

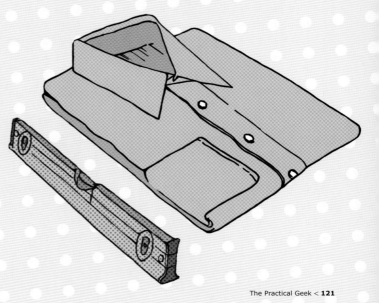

How to Care for Your Knitwear

Quality comes at a certain price, but does not necessarily need to be preciously treated. With a degree of care and attention all merino wool and cotton garments can be machine washed and will continue to look good and last well for many years to come. These top tips for extra-fine merino wool knitwear come from **John Smedley**, who have been manufacturing some of the world's finest knitwear since 1784. The body panels and sleeves of the wool and cotton garments are linked together by hand, stitch for stitch, to create the impeccable neat seams which remain one of the hallmarks of real luxury knitwear. After knitting, the garments are scoured or washed using water from John Smedley's underground springs – this is a crucial stage in the manufacturing process and gives the garments their characteristic "soft handle". Additional processes render the pieces shrink resistant and machine washable, a unique feature considering such delicate techniques are applied.

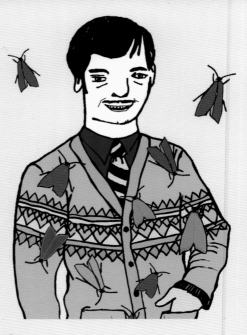

1 Remove surface soiling by gentle brushing; this will help lift the stain later on.

2 Treat stains immediately with cold water and blot dry with a clean cloth, never paper.

3 Air wool after wearing by laying the garment flat as this helps to get rid of odours.

4 Always try to store lightweight wool folded and allow breathing space around the garment.

5 Clean your garments before storing. The dreaded moths seemingly love top-quality fibres, but they are actually feeding off body oils and dirt, not the actual fibre.

6 Use natural remedies to combat moth attack – the old treatments perform the best and smell great too. Cloves, lavender, rosemary and thyme, orange peel and cedar can all help deter the munchers. Never put the ingredients in direct contact with the knitwear, however; instead tie them in a gauze bag and hang in your cupboard or closet. It is worth noting that as we have ditched carpets in favour of floorboards, the moths no longer have floor coverings to attack, so are more inclined toward your clothes.

7 Try to rest your wool garment between wearings (if you can bear to!). A full 24 hours allows the natural fibres to spring back and preserves their natural resilience.

8 Turn the garment inside out to protect the outer surface, then wash in a cool (30°C/86°F) cycle. Merino wool has natural self-cleaning properties so you don't have to wash so often and this in turn protects the environment. For stains and soiling, cold-soak prior to washing to loosen dirt and prevent it from fixing permanently with hot water.

9 Use a mild, non-biological detergent. Biological enzymes eat away at natural fibres, causing longterm damage.

10 Dry flat, or outside on a good-quality clothesline on a windy day (the fibre almost returns to its natural habitat!).

11 Use a gentle, warm iron with steam to just return the shape – though if worn straight from the clothes line, no ironing is necessary.

12 Wash dark and lights separately, keep the temperatures low and never hang black or dark colours on the washing line in bright sunshine. Natural sunlight is the best bleaching agent – perfect to keep your whites white!

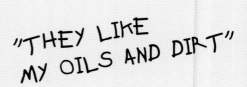

"THEY LIKE MY OILS AND DIRT"

How to Care for Your Leather Jacket

The leather jacket is an investment piece and not something you should or could afford to replace often. Quality leather will improve with age but there are still things you can do to keep your leather jacket looking its best.

★ DON'T store your leather jacket in a plastic bag.

★ DON'T place on a metal hanger – the kind you get from the dry-cleaners – as this will ruin the shape.

★ DO allow your jacket to air-dry if it becomes wet.

★ DON'T use a blowdryer or hand-dryer as a quick fix-it option to dry off the coat.

★ DO try to dry-clean your jacket at least once a year to ensure longevity and freshness.

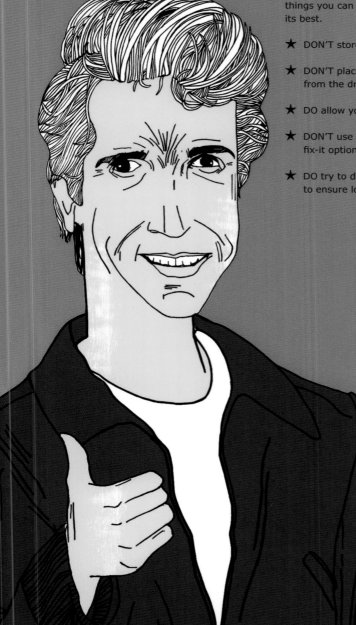

How to Store Your Neckties

A tie can make or break a look, so own a good selection. Plain, patterned and club ties in various widths and textures are good to have on standby for any occasion or outfit. Caring for your ties does not have to be expensive or tedious and a little knowledge can extend their lives. Here's the The Chic Geek's advice on how to store them.

① Handle with care. Ties, especially silk ones, have a fairly fragile shape. Pulling too hard on one end of a tie can result in stretched fabric, buckled stitches and a misshapen appearance.

② Wearing the same tie for too many days in a row can deepen the wrinkles and creases caused by normal wear. Two consecutive days is the maximum.

③ Although many people store ties by hanging them over a tie rack, this is not the best way as creases can develop. Instead, store your ties in loose rolls by rolling each one around with your hand. If a tie has creases, hang it for a couple of days to help the wrinkles fall out, but don't forget to roll it up and put it away afterward! Never store your ties with the knots still in them.

④ Remove creases with a special hand-steamer. Some tie manufacturers recommend you steam out the wrinkles with a steamer every couple of months in order to preserve a like-new appearance. Avoid ironing if you can – many tie connoisseurs complain that ironing a tie flattens out the rolled edges.

⑤ If you opt for dry cleaning, be sure to choose a cleaner who specializes in dry cleaning ties, particularly if you need to have a stain removed.

How to Tie a Bow-tie

We will take it as read that you know how to tie a standard necktie, so I'm going to talk about tying a bow-tie here. Knowing how to tie a bow-tie is a bit like learning to juggle; it's a skill that you'll probably not use very often but it's nice to know you can do it. Here are the steps, but if you're struggling, look on YouTube or elsewhere on the Internet for a demonstration video that will make it easy to understand.

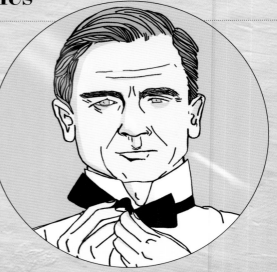

① Adjust the tie's length so it fits your neck; they are usually easily adjustable. Sizes are usually marked.

② Lift up your shirt collar and put the tie around your neck so the ends hang down at the front. One end should hang about 3.5 to 5 cm (1½ to 2 inches) lower than the other.

③ Bring the longer end across, behind and over the short end to form a simple knot. Pull snugly around your neck.

④ Fold the shorter end of the bow-tie at the widest point, where the hourglass shape begins to narrow, to form a bow shape. The bow shape should be in front. Hold the bow in a horizontal position at your neck.

⑤ Bring the longer end of the bow tie over and in front of the shorter end.

⑥ Fold the longer end at the widest point to form a second bow and then bring this bow under the first bow.

⑦ Tuck it into the space behind the first bow.

⑧ Adjust the shape of the two bows.

Keep trying until it looks good. Practise makes perfect! It will never look as tidy or neat as a pre-tied or clip-on, but that's the whole point – it gives the bow-tie character.

How NOT to Wear a Tie

Raphael le Masne de Chermont, the founder of the Mandarin Collar Society and executive chairman of **Shanghai Tang**, gives us the Mandarin Collar Society manifesto. The Mandarin Collar Society was inaugurated by Shanghai Tang to promote the mandarin collar around the world. There are specific Mandarin Collar Society counters at Shanghai Tang flagship stores worldwide. The Mandarin Collar Society believes:

★ Neckties are often discarded when men reach a certain level of success and achievement.

★ Neckties are the bearers of bad news: they show and tell the wearer when he has gained weight.

★ Neckties have no obvious function other than as soup bibs and something for adversaries to grab in a fight.

★ Neckties waste time, encourage tardiness and contribute to trillions of lost work hours.

★ Neckties are increasingly uncomfortable as the Earth's temperature rises because of global warming.

★ Neckties are just fancy choke collars to impose conformity, invite enslavement and remind the wearer that his superiors have him by the neck.

★ Neckties present health risks, choke off the oxygen supply, contribute to glaucoma and are immediately removed in medical emergencies.

★ Neckties require expensive dry cleaning and waste money that could otherwise be spent on necessities, such as golf clubs.

★ Neckties cannot be worn with today's ultimate style statement, the mandarin collar.

How to Look After Your Leather Shoes

Quality leather shoes are an investment and should be respected as such. One of Northampton's finest shoemakers, **Church's**, here tells us how to look after them. Church's was founded in 1873 by Thomas Church and his three sons Alfred, William and Thomas Jr, who could count on family experience in the production of handmade men's shoes dating back to 1675.

"Leather soles are a natural product and, as such, are breathable and flexible. Because of their porous nature it is essential that they are not worn in consistently wet conditions. It is suggested that your shoes should be worn in dry conditions first, which will harden the sole and lessen the penetration of water.

"Before you wear your shoes, polish them to give them that additional coating. Your leather uppers will require regular cleaning and polishing with the appropriate wax polish or shoe cream in a colour that is closest to your shoes; if in doubt, always select a neutral wax.

"It is recommended that you thoroughly clean your shoes, removing all mud with a soft damp cloth or welt brush. For suede leathers, remove all surface dirt with a rubber suede brush and take care to avoid getting them wet or damp. At this point remove any stains using a proprietary cleaner or by rubbing the suede very gently with fine sandpaper or an emery cloth.

"Allow the leather to dry out at room temperature away from hot pipes, radiators or fires; this will allow the leather to retain its original features. It is advisable after cleaning to use a pair of shoetrees. The trees will help retain the shoes original shape, particularly when drying, and prevent them from creasing.

"Apart from the final appearance, the purpose of polishing your shoes is to build up and maintain an even film over the surface of the leather. This will preserve and enhance its natural beauty, protect the surface and minimize the risk of staining due to severe wetting of the shoe.

"Church's always recommend you use a shoe horn when putting your shoes on; this will prevent damage to the backs. When storing shoes, retain the shoe-box that came with them, ensure shoes are dry and simply store in cloth bags in the box. We would advise that to prolong the life of your shoes, you should alternate pairs daily to allow your shoes time to rest."

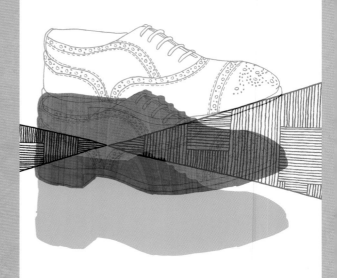

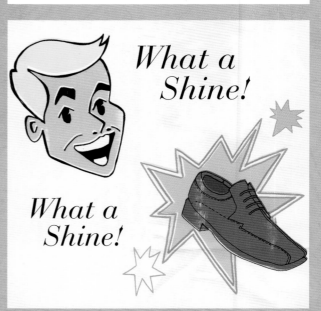

What a Shine!

What a Shine!

How to Shine Your Shoes

Cherry Blossom, the first and now the only UK manufacturer of shoe polish, shows us how to really get our shoes shining. The iconic "one penny tin" with its original butterfly twist opener was introduced in 1907, as was the name "Cherry Blossom Boot Polish".

1 It is most important that you start with perfectly clean shoes. Do this by wiping the shoes with a damp cloth, then spray with a cleaner such as Cherry Blossom Premium's Universal cleaner.

2 Shake well, hold upright and spray. Keep the can 10 to 15 cm (4 to 6 inches) away from the shoes and spray a even amount covering all of the leather.

3 Use a soft cloth or soft-haired shoe brush to work the foam into the solid areas.

4 Wait 10 seconds and wipe the dirt away with a clean cloth.

5 Allow the shoes to dry at room temperature.

6 Use a premium leather cream suitable for all colours so there's no need to colour match to your shoes. This nourishes and protects the leather. Using a sponge, sparingly spread the cream all over the shoe.

7 Work the cream in a circular motion over the entire surface of the shoe. Always make sure you work the cream into all the crevices and cracks in the leather. Leave to dry for 3 minutes.

8 Take a traditional soft-haired shoe brush and buff the shoes in a left-to-right motion to remove any excess polish. Voilà, what a shine!

How to Look After Your Glasses & Sunglasses

① Never put them on the top of your head – this stretches them out.

② Don't leave them in the sun or in your car. Plastic frames will distort in the heat and lose their shape.

③ Always store them in their hard case when not in use.

④ Good eyewear needs maintenance. Go to the opticians every three to six months to have the screws tightened, nose pads cleaned or changed and the glasses adjusted.

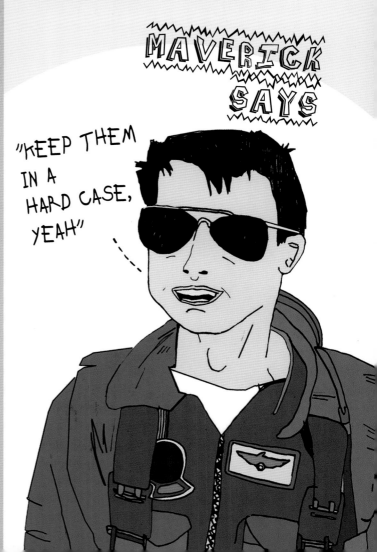

MAVERICK SAYS

"KEEP THEM IN A HARD CASE, YEAH"

How to Choose Glasses

Sunglasses and spectacles are furniture for the face. A good pair of glasses will enhance your appearance and suit your personality. Styles come and go, evolving to suit the day's fashion but there are a few rules to follow regarding the choice of frames dictated by the shape of your face and colouring.

★ Try on lots of different pairs even if you initially don't think they're your style. It's good to find out what you don't like or doesn't suit you to focus yourself.

★ Take a patient friend along for their opinion. The optician is usually pretty good at this too.

★ It sounds obvious but make sure that your eyes are positioned in the middle of the lenses. If your eyes are close together, avoid larger frames.

★ Your eyebrows should align with the top bar of the glasses.

★ Choose smaller frames if you have facial hair such as a beard. Large frames will further mask your features.

★ Avoid wearing frames that have a similar shape to your face. Choose frames in a different cut to your face shape.

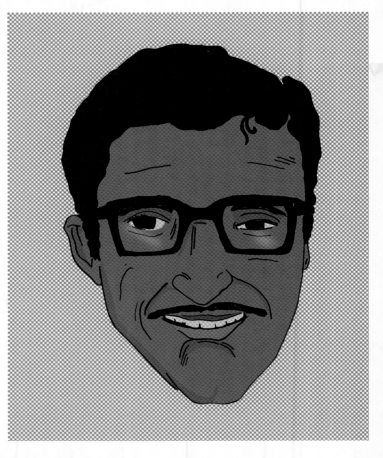

★ It's all about proportions. Stick with small frames if you have a small head. Make sure your glasses are no any wider than the widest part of your face.

★ Oval faces are egg-shaped and balanced on top and bottom, so can support any type of frame.

★ Frames made of thin metal soften the angular look of a square face, which has a wide forehead and cheeks plus an angular chin.

★ Avoid heavy branding or large logos.

★ Be practical. If you are a bit heavy-handed or want your glasses to last, get a more robust frame.

★ Make a long, thin face seem wider and shorter with larger frames in round or triangular shapes. Or try a wide, rectangular shape. Frames that have colour, width or embellishment near the sides will also broaden your face.

Travel Basics

Ideally you would take your whole wardrobe and have a valet to pack and unpack when you get there but let's get real: the amount we can take away is getting smaller because of airline costs so we all need to be economical with style. Travel is a great opportunity to think about the way you dress, it's like a crash-diet for your over-blown wardrobe and makes you more inventive with what you have.

★ The best place to start is to think about the events you'll attend while you're away; for example, you might be going to a business meeting or a friend's wedding. Plan each outfit individually right down to the socks and shoes you are going to wear. These items go in the definite pile.

★ Now, think about activities. Are you going swimming or to the beach while you're away? Add these items.

★ Next up are the basics: underwear, socks, T-shirts and jeans. Take underwear for each day plus one, just in case!

★ Finally, any room left can be used for extra items. Choose a palette of neutrals so most combinations work together. Also check the weather forecast: if it's really hot, there's not much point in taking too many sweaters or jeans.

★ To continue looking stylish while you're away, add accessories. This is where the highlights are. Scarves, ties, belts and glasses will add touches of style and won't take up too much room.

★ For larger items like coats or jackets, wear these on the plane or train so you don't have to pack them.

★ Streamline your grooming bag. Choose products with a dual function; for example, a body wash that is also a shampoo or a moisturizer with sun protection. If you're only going for a few days, take the very basics.

★ Pack a simple outfit in take-on hand luggage, just in case your suitcase gets lost. Hand luggage should also be used for anything fragile, expensive, medical or things that cannot be easily replaced.

How to Pack a Suitcase

The main rule is try not to overpack or underpack, so things don't get too crushed but are firm enough not to move around. Here are The Chic Geek's top tips.

1 First, make sure the suitcase is clean and smells fresh and clean. Mark the case or ensure it is distinctive enough so there is no confusion at the airport carousel.

2 Fasten everything on your clothes – buttons, zips, etc. – so garments keep their shape better and don't catch on each other.

3 Lie trousers on top of each other before you put them in the case and fold them once over each other.

4 Lie shirts on top of each other and then fold the arms in and roll the body up toward the neck; this saves space and prevents creases.

5 Stuff socks into your shoes to save on space.

6 Place shoes in shoe bags and arrange them along the border of your suitcase.

7 Store toiletries in plastic bags to protect everything else from leaks.

8 Put your nightwear at the top so you don't have to dig around for it if it's late when you get there.

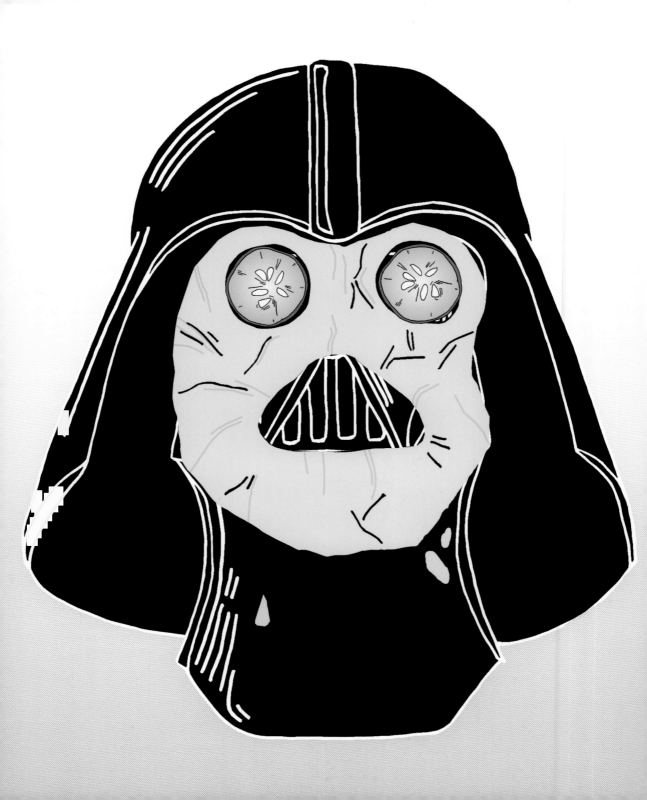

5 Grooming for Geeks

Just as you look after your wardrobe, it's equally important to take care of yourself; it's part and parcel of looking stylish. A clear complexion and glossy hair are essential components of looking your best no matter how well you are dressed.

The foundations of looking good are a healthy and balanced lifestyle – eating well, de-stressing and getting enough exercise. A grooming regime is the icing on top and has become an integral part of the modern male's armoury. From the follicle on his head to his pedicured toe, today's man has more products and treatments at his disposal than ever before. Try not to be blinded by science; instead ask your hair stylist, dermatologist, doctor or pharmacist any questions you have, no matter how obvious or ridiculous you think they are, as it's the only way to learn and to de-mystify the technical lingo.

Be open to trying new treatments and products that will help to enhance and relax you, too. Men are respected today for caring for themselves – grooming is not a vain exercise or a slippery slope into a full face of make-up but an area where the individual can discover what works for him and what makes him feel and look better. For some men this may be just a dab of moisturizer, for others it could be a little more complicated. It will take a bit of experimentation but the following few pages will give you a helping hand when it comes to looking after all the areas of your body – skin, teeth, hair, hands and feet – as well as information on staying healthy in the sun and smelling as good as you look.

Protecting Your Skin from the Sun

Dr Tom Mammone, Clinique's Executive Director of Skin Physiology and Pharmacology, gives some advice on protecting your skin.

"Start simply. Clean the dirt from your skin with a great soap and exfoliate – you'd never paint a wall without prepping it first. Then enhance; put something on your skin that is protective. Always use a facial product that provides UVA (these are the penetrating rays that cause deeper skin damage) and UVB (rays that give you wrinkles) protection. Reduce processed sugars in your diet, too. A sugary diet and sun damage combined can seriously damage the skin."

Suntan Lotions

When it comes to suntan lotions and creams it isn't so much about the factor number (though choose one according to your skin type) as it is about application.

★ Always apply in quantity and evenness.

★ Protect all the prime exposure areas, such as the tops of feet, the ears, etc.

★ Reapply every two hours regardless of the factor number as some lotions can break down after two hours and it is not worth taking the risk. Sweat can also dissolve the cream on the skin.

★ Choose a product specifically formulated to protect the face, which is always exposed. The formula will be specifically targeted for thinner facial skin.

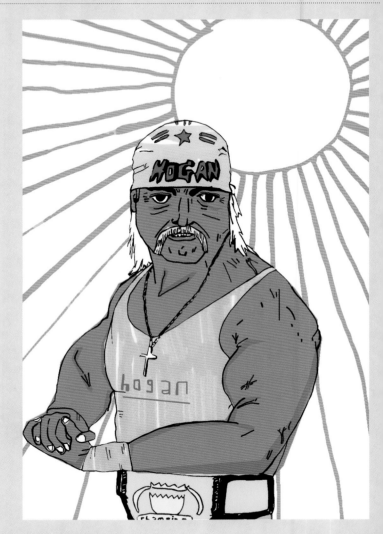

Anti-Ageing Ingredients

Father Time may march on but, like Dorian Gray, who wants to show it? The world of "anti-ageing" can be a bit like the Emperor's New Clothes with so many different claims and promises from various companies about their products. Luckily, as men we have thicker and oilier skin than women, which helps us age better; nevertheless there are still things we can do to help ourselves. The key is "prevention rather than cure". This is a longterm commitment so you can't expect results overnight; you need to keep your skin looking younger when you have youth on your side rather than trying to turn back time later on. There are many new anti-ageing products specifically aimed at men which offer to give your skin a bit of extra help in its old age and here are some key ingredients to look out for in products.

Alpha-Hydroxy Acids (AHAs) These anti-ageing ingredients are commonly used for their exfoliating properties. They also provide a skin-tightening effect that diminishes fine lines.

Antioxidants These are substances that may protect cells from the damage caused by unstable molecules known as free radicals.

Beta-Hydroxy Acids (Salicylic Acid) This gentler form is for those with sensitive skin and since it has the ability to penetrate deeply, it's also good for oily or acne-prone skin. It offers the same exfoliating qualities along with the ability to unclog pores.

Caviar Loaded with protein, vitamins and minerals, and with a cell format similar to human skin, caviar helps speed up the natural production of collagen. In time this plumps and thickens the skin to give a younger, firmer appearance.

Coenzyme Q10 (Ubiquinone) This antioxidant may help to repair skin damaged by the elements and improve collagen production.

Green Tea Contains powerful antioxidants that will destroy free radicals.

Peptides Anti-ageing benefits stem from their power to stimulate collagen, which is responsible for maintaining the texture and elasticity of our skin.

Sirtuins These are the new longevity proteins (resveratrol, found in grapes and red wine, is a sirtuin activator), which increase the skin cell's life span.

Suncreen A high level of UVA protection will protect against UVA radiation, associated with ageing effects such as wrinkles.

Vitamin A (Retinol, Tretinoin and Retinyl Palmitate) In various formulations the vitamin has been shown to reduce fine lines and pores.

Vitamin C (ascorbic acid) Topical creams are proven to help control wrinkles and fine lines.

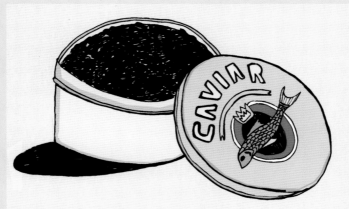

How to Look After Your Skin

When it comes to your skin, you get out what you put in. What is usually bad for the inside, such as smoking and unhealthy eating, will be reflected on the outside. A healthy, balanced diet and drinking plenty of water rewards you and your skin. Too much partying and boozing will be reflected in breakouts and dehydration.

Male skin is generally thicker than female skin and because of higher testosterone levels, men are more prone to oiliness and acne breakouts. Men also have to contend with rough, dry textured skin due to daily aggression from regular shaving, which increases the skin's sensitivity and decreases elasticity. Below are a few things we can do to limit the toil our playboy lifestyles have on our skin.

★ Reduce stress. Easier said than done, but take some time out to relax and unwind.

★ Eat dark leafy greens such as broccoli and spinach, which contain antioxidants that cleanse your skin from the inside. Superfoods such as berries are also great for the skin.

★ Limit sugar and high glycemic index carbohydrates (carbs that break down quickly and elevate your blood sugar level) like watermelon, rice and heavily processed foods.

★ Don't smoke; it ages the skin.

★ Do not use soap. It has an alkaline pH and strips your skin of natural acidity, leaving skin dehydrated. Don't use anything that makes your skin feel tight after rinsing.

★ Always protect your skin from the sun. Think "daylight" rather than "sunlight"; even when it's overcast, you still need to protect your skin.

★ Exfoliate a couple of times a week. Most products contain granulated pumice, salicylic acid, alpha-hydroxy acid and beta hydroxy acid, all which help slough off dead skin cells. Don't overdo it or use anything too harsh, though. The sandpaper-like sensation of some facial scrubs might feel effective, but can be traumatic for your skin. Use exfoliators with rounded granules.

★ Be gentle with your skin, particularly around delicate areas like the eyes.

★ Protect from air pollution. A daily moisturizer containing antioxidants and SPF will offer some protection.

Your Skincare Regime

Take a tip from the girls and try the classic three-step rule: cleanse, tone and moisturize. Choose products targeted specifically for your skin type: dry, oily, combination, sensitive or normal. Good skin maintenance can improve the tone and appearance, reduce wrinkles or clogged pores and increase confidence too.

① To remove everyday dirt, pollution and oil, use a multi-action face wash or cream or gel cleanser morning and night. Cream cleansers are good for drier skins while gels suit oiler skin.

② Follow with an everyday toner or use an exfoliator two to three times a week for this stage. A gentle toner will clear away any remaining dead skin cells and leave your skin looking and feeling fresh, while an exfoliator works at a deeper level to slough away skin.

③ Moisturize with an SPF product. This adds a protective layer to your skin to guard against environmental damage and puts moisture back into your skin.

Masks for Men

And you thought masks were just for *The Phantom of the Opera*. Every man loves a sly pamper session but remember what happens in the bathroom stays in the bathroom. Applying a clay mask is a great way to draw out hidden oils and grime, tighten pores and reduce blackheads, while moisturizing cream masks hydrate drier skins and peel-off or exfoliating masks deeply cleanse by lifting off the top layer of dead skin cells. Look at the benefits of each type before choosing one that suits you. Most masks should only be used once a week.

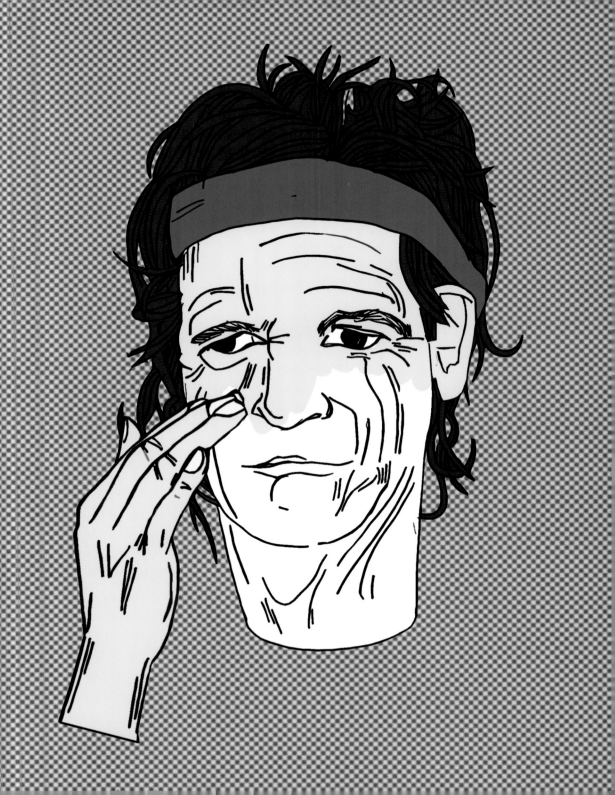

Body Care

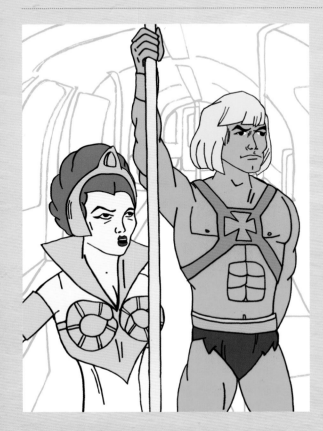

★ Dry your armpits well before adding anti-perspirant or deodorant to reduce the amount of staining or yellowing on your clothes.

★ When it comes to your mouth, drink plenty of water and brush your teeth, tongue and gums regularly. Using a mouthwash may also help. A tongue scraper will remove some of the bacteria at the back of your tongue.

★ Deal with the root cause of any body odour or breath problem, rather than trying to mask it. Breath mints and strong deodorants won't deal with a longterm problem, so visit the doctor or dentist to get advice.

★ Some people perspire more than others; if you need to shower more than once a day or change your clothes more often, then that's what you must do. You'll feel fresher and more confident as a result.

★ Wear undergarments or clothes that have been directly in contact with your body only once and wash everything else regularly. If a garment is difficult to wash, make sure you wear a washable layer in between you and it.

★ If you've spent time and money on a great quality fragrance, don't add on cheap spray-on deodorants; go un-scented underneath.

★ Men often fail to wash and scrub their feet and to clean between the toes. If your feet are a problem, devote more time to them. Men with foot odour problems should invest in products such as sprays and powders, which can eliminate the smell and reduce sweating.

★ Some types of shoe will make your feet smell more than others; often it's down to the manmade materials or getting your shoes wet. Never wear the same shoes every day; instead alternate so you can give them a chance to dry out and air.

You want to smell as good as you look. Personal hygiene is very much that, personal, and you need to find a routine that works for you.There's nothing more disconcerting than worrying that you have bad breath or body odour. Face up and ask a trusted friend. They probably won't tell you until you mention it, but if you suspect something, what's the harm in asking? At least then you can do something about it.

Men usually have more body hair that traps bacteria, dirt and odours. It is the bacteria built up on the skin and within hair follicles that smells and not the sweat. Do the basics – like washing your body and brushing your teeth – well. When it comes to washing, men have a habit of soaking themselves in hot water and barely drying before dressing. This results in the body becoming a breeding ground for bacteria that causes you to smell and also can stain your clothes. Here are some tips on being your fragrant self.

The Perfect Smile

Dr Anjali Rajah of NW Smiles gives her tips on how to look after your teeth below. Without sounding obvious, it is important to brush twice daily, floss and use a mouthwash once a day. Try using tongue detoxers to keep your mouth fresh and healthy too.

★ Use a mid-priced electric toothbrush to clean teeth well and keep gums healthy. Electric toothbrushes are recommended over hand toothbrushes, as they rotate much faster (5000–7000 revolutions/minute). All-round electric toothbrushes allow a much more effective clean. Most electric toothbrushes also have timers on them to indicate the correct length of time for brushing, which should be two minutes.

★ Place the head of the toothbrush 45 degrees into the angle of the gum, use only gentle pressure (excessive force can lead to gum recession), then after a few seconds move the brush onto the surface of the tooth to give it a good clean too. Some more sophisticated electric toothbrushes have pressure sensors built in so the movement alters if too much pressure is applied onto the surface of your teeth and gums.

★ You should brush for two minutes each time, morning and night (allow 30 seconds for each quadrant in your mouth). Use a slim line of toothpaste for adults, a pea-size amount for children.

★ Always choose brush heads that have dye indicators, which fade over a period of time (three to four months), indicating a new head is required. Make sure you replace your brushes and dental tools every three months. This is because the bristles will splay over time and are then not so effective at cleaning.

★ Regular flossing is essential to maintain a healthy smile. Flossing allows removal of plaque which builds up between the teeth, however most people dislike flossing due to the difficulty in access, especially at the back of the mouth. Hummingbirds are small battery-operated flossers which vibrate, making flossing in between teeth easier. The shape also allows better access to all areas of the mouth.

★ Avoid drinking red wine and instead opt for rosé or white. Avoid drinking black tea and coffee and always add milk to protect teeth from staining. Dark herbal teas may also stain, so watch out for these drinks too!

★ Avoid whitening toothpastes; some may be abrasive and can result in teeth sensitivity. Instead have your teeth whitened professionally at a dental surgery. Home-whitening kits use gel placed in trays; the trays need to be worn for 10 to 14 days to see the best results.

★ Use a whitening pen, such as BriteSmile To Go Teeth, after drinking heavy -staining beverages. It's a neat, portable teeth whitener that's perfect for men and women with busy lifestyles and hassle-free compared to using awkward teeth trays.

★ For an isolated dark tooth, you could also have a composite or porcelain veneer fitted.

★ Finally, visit your dentist every 6 to 12 months for a check-up and clean to ensure your mouth and oral hygiene is maintained and your teeth and gums are kept in good condition at all times.

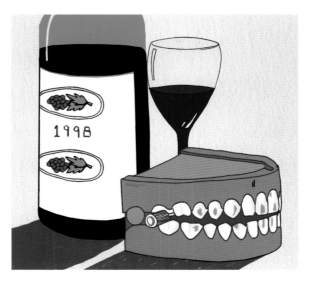

How to Shave When You're Prone to Blemishes

Jessica Bailey-Woodward, representative of **Proactiv®** skincare solutions in the UK, offers some pointers on shaving for those with acne problems.

"One of the biggest problems facing men who suffer from blemishes is shaving. This can be painful, frustrating and may also lead to a number of problems. The following guidelines will help.

"It is essential that you wash your face before you shave to make the skin supple and soft, then apply shaving cream or foam to areas on your face that are blemish-free. Always try and use a fresh, disposable razor with each shave. Check your skin before you start so you're aware of where the blemishes are and can avoid them. Unless a blemish is large and sore, you should be able to shave right over it without causing further infection.

Alternatively, consider using an electric shaver as this may be more comfortable and is less likely to scratch your blemishes. However, if you do stick to water shaving, make sure all the products you use on your face are oil- and alcohol-free.

★ Even if you have oily skin, you must remember to moisturize. This is because when skin becomes dry and begins to lose its delicate balance, it will compensate by producing even more oil. Moisturizing keeps your skin nourished and healthy, not oily.

★ Fake it, don't bake it. Sun exposure can be bad for blemishes, as tanning stimulates both peeling and oil production simultaneously – and this is a recipe for clogged pores.

★ Don't overuse moisturizer and apply lotions sparingly – all you need is enough to lightly cover the entire surface of the skin where needed. Too much will just clog pores.

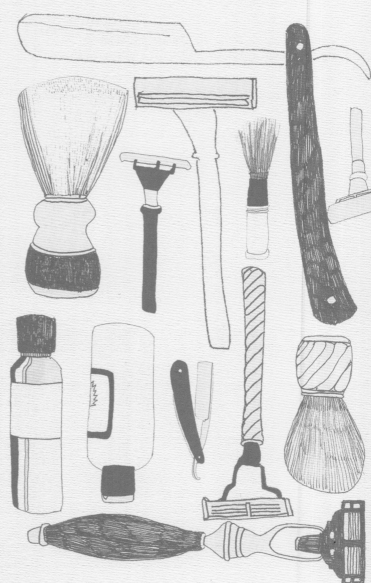

How to Get the Perfect Shave

Do not shave the moment you get up; you will achieve a closer shave if you wait for at least 20 minutes to allow the facial muscles to tighten. The advice below comes from **Truefitt & Hill** in London, the world's oldest barbershop, with over 200 years of experience. They are currently barbers and Royal Warrant holders to HRH The Duke of Edinburgh and have international outposts in Chicago, Toronto and Las Vegas.

① Prepare. The key to the perfect shave is to prepare your skin. If possible, shave during or just after a hot shower. Alternatively, soften whiskers with a hot, damp towel, pressing over the contours of your face for 20 seconds. The heat and moisture helps soften the beard and prepares skin for the shave.

② Apply a pre-shave oil. Designed to protect the skin from the razor blade, the oil softens the whiskers of the beard and helps the blade glide smoothly, so reducing irritation and nourishing the skin. Work a little oil into the face and beard before applying shaving cream.

③ Apply shaving cream. Using a shaving brush helps to create a rich lather and lifts each individual whisker, coating the whiskers and helping to give the smoothest shave possible.

④ Shave with or across the grain of your beard, not against it. Shaving against the grain is the main cause of irritation and razor burn. Rinse the razor regularly and use a good-quality blade, remembering to replace the blade often. A dull blade is a common cause of razor burn and irritation.

⑤ Moisturize. After shaving, rinse your face with cold water to close the pores of the skin. Pat dry and apply a soothing and moisturizing aftershave balm.

How to Trim Your Beard

While everyone experiences hair growth at different rates, you should typically allow the hair to grow in length for around four to six days. Ensure that your electric clipper has graded numbers and a half setting to allow for some flexibility in choosing your preferred length. The grades refer to the length of the hair in millimeters; for example, grade 1 means the hair will be cut to between 1–3 mm in length whereas grade 2 represents between 2–6 mm in length. Alternatively, your clipper may be set in inches with a variety of settings – such as from $\frac{1}{16}$–$\frac{1}{2}$ inches – and attachments.

① **Do make certain that you start with a dry beard**. If you're unsure how short you would like your beard to be, it's best to start trimming with a higher clipper grade. You can then repeat the process with a lower grade, if you wish. In cases where the thickness of the beard differs on various parts of the face, it's best to use a short grade on thicker areas such as the chin or moustache area, and a longer grade on the thinner areas to achieve an even finish.

② **When you are happy with the length**, take some time tidying up your beard. Set your clipper on 0 and remove the clipper guard, if you have been using one. The teeth should be closed. Tilting your head back slightly, use the flat side of your clipper to create a line from left to right above the Adam's apple. Use your own discretion but try not to take the line too high or too low. To create a natural finish to the beard, trim the neck area with the clippers on a grade lower than you used to trim the bulk of the beard. You can apply a small amount of shaving oil into the beard when finished to ensure it looks shiny and healthy.

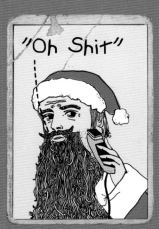

"Oh Shit"

How to Wax "Downstairs"

Carleigh Rayner, training manager of **Strip** boutique (*see also* page 171), gives us a step-by-step guide to waxing our "male intimate areas". Strip has a Manifico treatment room created especially for men, offering a virtually pain-free waxing experience.

1 Waxing will give you the best results on the male intimate areas and removes hair from the root meaning it will last for approximately four weeks. The hair in the area to be waxed should be at least 4 mm long ($\frac{1}{6}$ in), so if you have been shaving or using hair removal creams allow the hair to grow back prior to waxing.

2 Book an appointment with a professional waxing therapist. It is vital that you do not attempt to wax yourself as the nether region is obviously very sensitive and any home job attempts may result in bruising, burning or raw skin.

3 Ensure your chosen salon uses hot wax for intimate areas. We would recommend Lycon's hot wax, as it is gentle and a pre-wax oil is used on the skin prior to the wax being applied; this means the wax only pulls directly on the hair and not the skin, resulting in a much less painful wax.

4 Ensure that the salon you book with has therapists fully trained in intimate male waxing – at least one year's salon experience to make sure you're in safe hands!

5 Some salons will have treatment rooms dedicated to men which also include a TV to help you relax during your treatment!

6 Do not trim the hair prior to your appointment as the therapist will do this for you. This will ensure the hair is the right length to wax and not too short.

7 Avoid any tanning for 48 hours prior to your appointment.

8 On the day of your wax do not apply any moisturizer to the area as this will result in the wax not working properly. Simply shower and have the area dry and clean.

9 Once in the treatment room with your therapist, feel free to discuss exactly what you would like done in the treatment. Do you want all the hair removed from the pubic area? Or would you like to leave some hair at the front and remove all of the hair from the underneath and bottom area? There are so many options!

10 To start the treatment the therapist will clean the area with an antibacterial lotion and then apply pre-wax oil. When removing hair from the scrotum, both the therapist and client will hold and support the area in order to keep the skin tight (the therapist will instruct you exactly where to hold). Between the pre-wax oil and supporting the area, there will be minimal pain as the skin will not move once the wax is removed. In order to wax the bottom area, you will usually be asked to bring your knees to your chest.

11 Depending on which salon you choose, it may also be possible to have dyeing done if you wish to leave some hair. Natural colours cover grey hairs or try fun colours like blue, red, pink, etc., if you're feeling outrageous!

12 Your therapist should give you home-care advice. It will be necessary for you to exfoliate the waxed area two to three times a week between waxes to avoid ingrown hairs either using a body scrub and/or an ingrown hair lotion.

13 Avoid public pools, saunas and gyms for at least 24 hours after your wax. As the pores will be open, you are more susceptible to picking up germs in this period.

14 Book your next wax now! For best results, wax every four weeks. This will result in a more comfortable wax and maximum hair-free time between waxes.

Great Eyebrows

Shavata has over 20 years' experience of creating the best brows in the business and currently runs a number of **Brow Studios** across the UK. Here are her top tips for men.

★ With men it depends on their individual personality. Are they a man's man, who prefers to keep it natural? Or are they more of a metrosexual man, who likes the manicured look? Regardless, all men should get their eyebrows trimmed on a regular basis and keep them tidy.

★ I personally think that men look better with manicured eyebrows and that there is no shame in a man plucking or threading. People often interpret shaped eyebrows as having a high distinctive arch but it doesn't have to be that way at all. If anything, you want people to look at you and not your eyebrows so the more natural they look, the better.

★ When done well, male brow-shaping can look really natural so half the time other people won't even know if you have had it done.

★ A basic shaping (between the brows and underneath the eyebrow) will simply make your eyebrows look clean and tidy. Male or female, a mono-brow is an absolute no-no! Just removing the hair from between the eyebrows makes all the difference to a man's appearance and will instantly draw attention to the eyes for all the right reasons.

★ To avoid mistakes, consult a professional for a first shaping, rather than take the situation into your own hands. They will give you a good starting shape, which you can then pluck and maintain yourself.

★ A brow tamer (clear mascara) is a great tool for keeping your eyebrows in place. Brow hairs grow in different directions so a quick slick of the tamer instantly gives a more uniform groomed look.

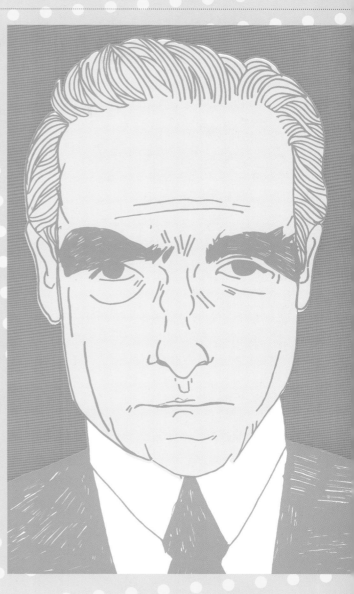

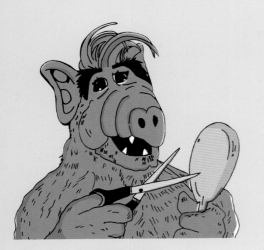

D I Y EYEBROWS:

① Always use natural daylight. No matter how hard you try, you will make mistakes in artificial light.

② Use both a hand mirror and a larger mirror when shaping eyebrows: a hand mirror for close-up plucking and a large one so you can sit back and look at both brows as you pluck, checking that they are even.

③ Eyebrows are sisters not twins, so never shape them separately. Using a good pair of quality stainless-steel tweezers, pluck a little at a time from both sides, always trying to keep to your natural shape so you are less likely to commit the cardinal sin of overplucking! Your eyebrows should start before the inner corner of the eyes, not after, so exercise some restraint.

④ Never pluck above the brow; this is your natural shape and you should never tweeze this area, as it won't grow back the same.

Looking After Your Hair

Like Samson, all our male strength is in our hair. Keeping your hair healthy and well-kempt, regardless of how much you've got left, is very important. Good-looking hair will make you look younger and more attractive.

★ No matter what the "science bit" of the adverts claims, nothing will repair split ends except a trim. If left uncut, they will continue to split higher up the shaft and can damage more of your hair.

★ Like any animal, the condition of your hair is often a reflection of your overall health. Eat well – oily fish, nuts, five-a-day fruit/vegetables, protein – exercise, drink plenty of water, get enough sleep and reduce stress in your life. Staying healthy also increases the rate of hair growth.

★ Wash your hair when it needs it, which will be different for everyone. Some men have to wash their hair every day while others get away with every other day, so find the routine that suits you. When washing your hair, be careful to avoid very hot water. It strips the essential oils from your hair and skin, which can lead to dullness and dryness.

★ Look for a shampoo and conditioner that is right for your hair type, and don't just chuck any old product on your head. Two-in-one products are mainly for use at the gym, which is fine but avoid using them too often.

★ When washing your hair, don't use too much shampoo – it really doesn't make your hair any cleaner the more bubbles you have.

★ Shampoo thoroughly, ensuring you cover all your hair in shampoo and gently massage the lather into the whole head of hair; do not rub. Use conditioner on the ends of your hair only, as applying it on the roots can make your hair greasy. And if you have very fine hair or are prone to greasy hair, don't condition more than once a week.

★ Pat your hair dry, as rubbing with a towel will damage it. Be warned: blowdrying and using straightening irons can dry out and damage the hair and scalp.

★ Finally, don't use too many styling products, chemical processes or colours on your hair. With prolonged use, they will weaken the hair shaft and will make your hair look tired. If you are going to sunbathe, make sure you protect your hair with a sunscreen product formulated for the hair and always wear a hat.

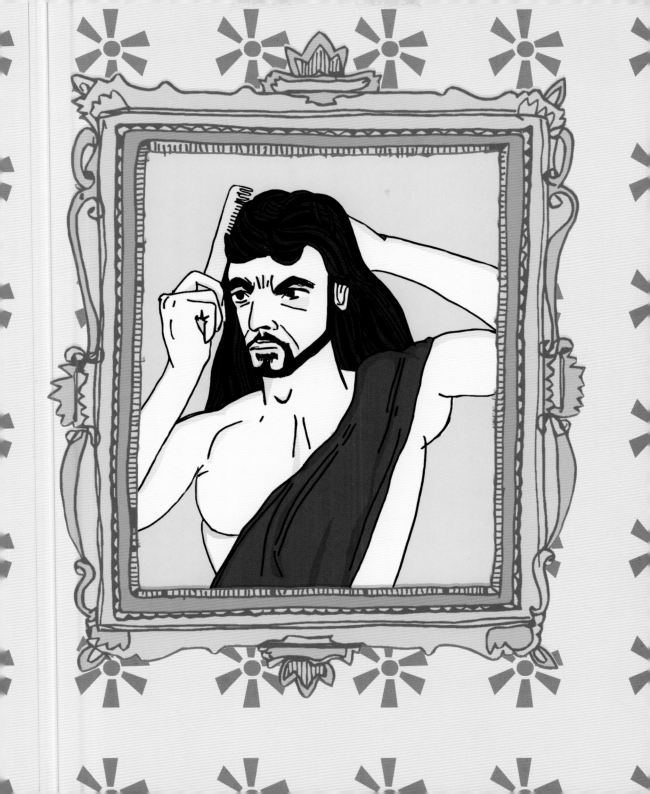

How to Get Great Hair

Marcio Oliveira, senior stylist at the **Jo Hansford**, London, advises on how to get great-looking hair, whatever the cut.

★ Remember, guys: rinse the hair very well to get out all of the shampoo and conditioner. The same applies to greasy scalps – regular shampooing with a suitable product will help to alleviate this problem.

★ A clean scalp, without flaking or dandruff, is essential. There are numerous products on the market to help cure or aid these problems. If you have a flaky or dry scalp, use a nutritious shampoo. For an itchy, flaky scalp or dandruff, apply Kérastase Bain Gommage. In both cases, Kérastase Lait Vital can be massage into the scalp after shampooing. If either of these symptoms persist, take professional advice.

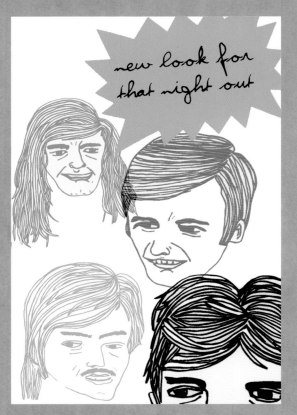

new look for that night out

★ If you have persistent scalp problems, take advice from your hairdresser or in extreme cases, a tricologist or doctor. Scalp problems can be caused by too much product used in the hair or not shampooing the product out sufficiently.

★ If you use a lot of products such as gels and waxes, it is a good idea to shampoo them out daily; normally one light shampoo in the shower will do. But with waxes or very heavy products, shampoo can be applied to the hair before the water and massaged in well, then add warm water and lather. Sometimes a second shampoo will be necessary.

★ For guys who are worried about losing their hair, I'm sorry but baldness is quite a common issue in men and it's hereditary so you can blame your parents! If you are experiencing this problem, you just have to accept it. Keep your hair cut short and neat, and go with it.

★ If you are lucky enough to have a clear scalp and good hair but you are starting to go grey, things can be done! You can subtly cover a few stray greys with a vegetable colour or a technique we use at Jo Hansford called a smudge, which is longer-lasting and a very effective coverage on a more permanent basis. If time is not a problem and your hair is short, high and lowlights are the way forward! But take advice from the colourist in your salon. Grey roots and a definite dark line are not good looks. There are products in your local pharmacy but still seek advice from a professional.

Styling Advice

★ Wear a style that suits you; following fashion is cool, but have your own image and look.

★ Find a product you can work with and do not be embarrassed to go for a new look.

★ Men tend to follow the female trend and our women clients like to have a style they can change, something casual in the daytime and a change of image for a party or night out.

How to Have and Maintain Dreadlocks

Johnnie Sapong, barber to the stars, gives the inside scoop on dreadlocks. Born in London and of Ghanaian origin, Sapong regularly works on top magazines as well as catwalk shows and for celebrity clients.

① It's best to work with some texture. If your hair is super straight, then it needs to be brushed, backcombed and teased to make it mat together before you begin. For new dreads, start with a steam treatment involving a hot towel and plastic cap.

② To form a section of dreadlocked hair, melt a little beeswax (available from a pharmacy or healthfood store), then attach to the hair while it is soft and molten; it will then harden up.

③ With new hair, continue with the twisting process. The hair needs to be re-twirled every eight weeks as it grows roughly 19 mm (¾ inch) a month. Our true belief – the Rastafari Movement – is that we don't cut the ends of the hair unless it keeps getting continually broken. We only cut our hair when somebody dies as a mark of respect and part of the life cycle.

④ After eight weeks, the hair will start to self-clean. Wear a hat, which supports the dreadlocks; we traditionally wear tam o'shanters.

Treatments for Dreads

Aloe vera sap is like a shampoo/conditioner; it oxygenates the scalp and cleanses the hair. It's hair food and acts as a soother and healer. You can get the aloe vera from a healthfood store or local farmer's market. To make a hair treatment, first break the plant up, place in a blender and make a pulp or liquid. Rub the aloe vera pulp into the hair, then wash this out; use a second application and leave in. Do not use detergents. Do this twice a month. Once a week, give the dreadlocks a warm water and then a cold water rinse.

For the scalp and roots of the hair, apply jojoba oil or carrot oil, which gives a slight fragrance or use lavender water when doing the cold rinse above.

Hands and Feet

Our hands and feet need regular maintenance. This doesn't have to mean costly or time-consuming manicures and pedicures, but do dedicate a small window of time to grooming. There is something very feminine feeling about the whole nail maintenance routine, but who cares? You're not doing this in front of an audience. Well-maintained hands and feet will show that you take pride in your appearance.

★ Don't bite your fingernails. I realize this is hard for those of you who do, but try and distract yourself. Trim any surplus growth little and often so you're less tempted to start biting.

★ Protect your hands as much as possible against abrasive detergents, gardening and frequent washing. It is important that you wear gloves when working around the house or garden, no matter how much of a woman you think you might look!

★ Use a mild soap if you wash your hands frequently, as the skin on the back of the hands is extremely delicate and can very quickly dry out.

★ Moisturize your hands regularly with a dedicated hand cream to keep them supple.

★ When it come to your feet, use a pumice stone on the heels, balls and sides of the feet and toes to help remove any dead skin cells before they are permitted to develop into unsightly dry and hard skin.

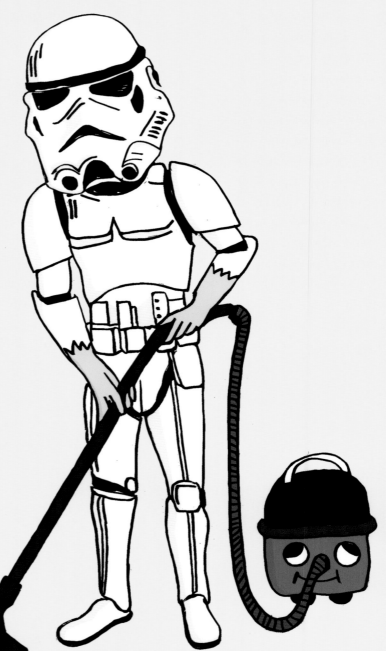

Home Manicure

① Before cutting your fingernails and toenails, clean the dirt and grime from underneath.

② To cut your nails, which you shouldn't rush, use a pair of nail scissors on your hands and special toenail clippers on your feet, as the nails are much thicker there and can twist and tear with nail scissors. Cut the toenail square across and not curved to prevent ingrowing nails. Don't cut too short either – after all, your nails are there for protection.

③ Now file your nails to give the desired, neat look. It is important to do your toenails as well as your fingernails because the sharp corners can tear through your socks and create holes. Always file in one direction only, toward the centre, keeping a square shape.

④ Push the cuticle skin back on your nails to promote healthy-looking nails. Do this when the skin is soft, such as after a bath, and use the blunt edge of a metal nail file or a wooden orange stick.

⑤ Finish by rubbing a special nail and cuticle oil, serum or cream into the bed of each nail.

You're now ready to shake hands with anybody!

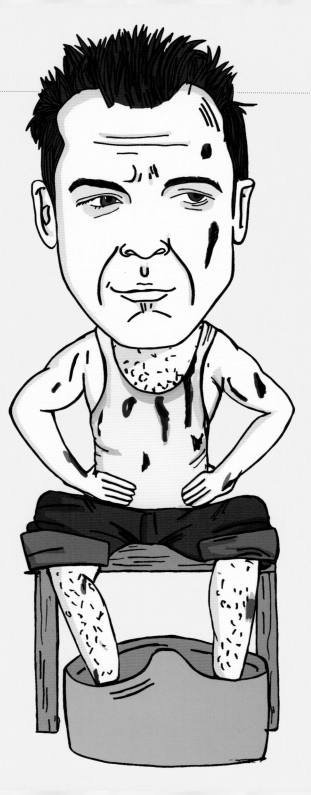

How to Get a Scent That Suits

Roja Dove is the world's sole Professeur de Parfums. He began his career at the French perfume house of Guerlain in Paris and now offers his expertise and experience as a consultant to some of the world's leading fragrance houses. Here is his advice.

★ Take note of the hype but don't be fazed by it. The image has nothing to do with the reality of perfume as there is no reality to perfume; it is the stuff of dreams.

★ Look everywhere… and I mean everywhere. Every store chases exclusives and you'll find smaller brands tucked away in a kind of perfume commune away from the major players – it's always worth checking them out for an undiscovered rarity that works for you.

★ Go it alone… never take a friend fragrance shopping. You have your agenda, they have one that's completely different. Something you like on yourself, they may think doesn't suit you at all. Contrary to what you may currently believe, this has little to do with how perfume develops on the skin. The idea that fragrances smell different on each individual is becoming a thing of the past; the more synthetics are used in the creation process, the less individual the fragrance will smell. A fragrance has to suit a wearer's personality.

★ Try lots… but how many can you try in one shopping day? More than you imagine if you take time. If you smell fragrances freshly sprayed, your nose will tire after the third one or so. This is due to the alcohol content, which works like an anaesthetic. It's a bit like drinking three gin and tonics and still expecting to have razor-sharp perception.

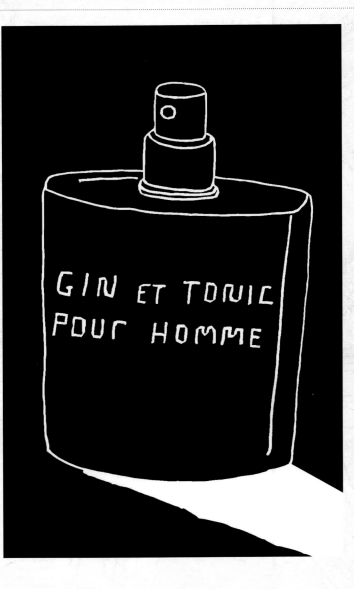

Testing a Scent

Smelling the perfume on paper on the "dry down" (when the perfume has settled and the alcohol has evaporated) means you can smell fragrances all day without fatigue. Testing on paper is the only sane way to try a fragrance. It's free from glues or binders and is as near to skin as it is possible to recreate; the only thing missing is the warmth of the skin, so breathe out very hard on the paper to warm it up before you inhale. Here's how.

① Always have unperfumed skin when going to buy a new scent, or the fragrances will fight against each other.

② Spray a few fragrances on blotter cards, turn them over to conceal the brand and then sniff them away from the perfumery department.

③ Smell them one at a time, comparing each one to the next, eliminating the one you like least of the two you're comparing, then continue the process until you have only one or a maximum of two fragrances left. Now turn the card to see which fragrance it is.

④ Go back to the counter and spray one, and only one, fragrance on your skin. And it shouldn't be a small squirt on your wrist. Spray it all over, then go away and sleep on it. A quick sniff is like flirting – just like a lover, it's only when you spend the night together that you know if the relationship is going to work out or not.

⑤ If you're still in love in the morning, buy it.

⑥ Isolate the "family" of perfumes (floral, chypre or oriental) you prefer by comparing and contrasting them. Sample different scents within the group you prefer to narrow down your selection.

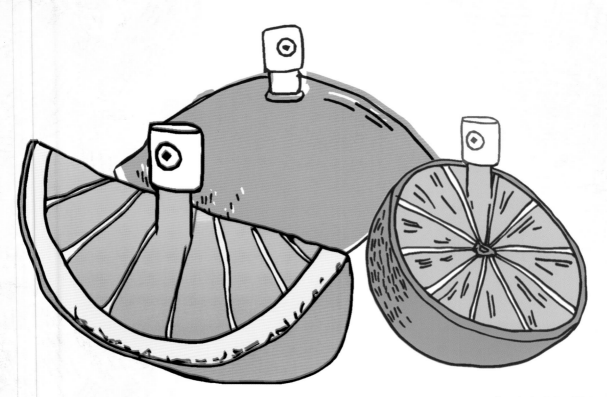

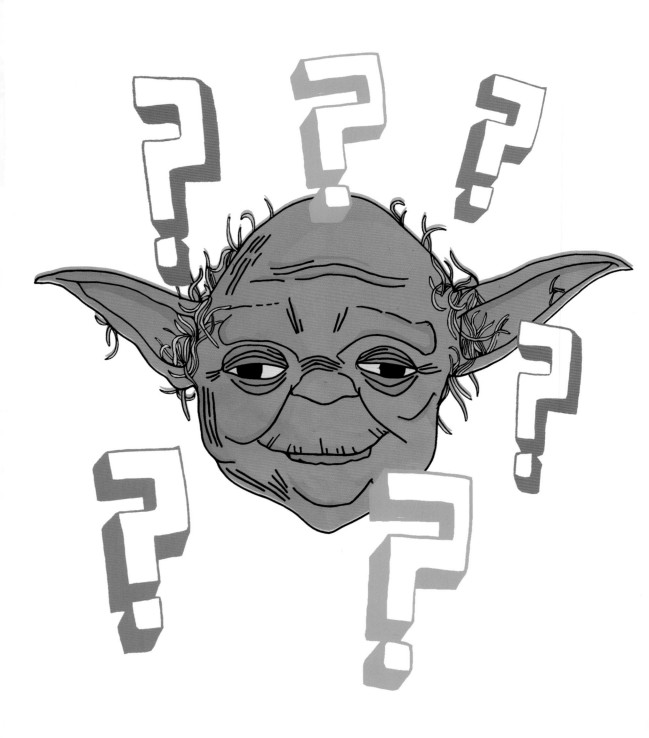

6 Ask the Geek

He's been there, done that and probably worn the T-shirt.
Now it's your chance to tap The Chic Geek's knowledge.
Ask the big man anything. His straight-talking, no-
nonsense approach will give you an honest answer based
on his knowledge of contemporary style and grooming.
This is where TheChicGeek.co.uk becomes interactive,
so make the most of it.

Want to find out what style of jean flatters you? Or
you have a practical fashion problem? Ask away. He's
here for all questions, no matter how trivial. The Chic
Geek likes to think of himself as that friend of yours who
knows a little bit more than you. He likes to share what
he discovers. The next few pages feature a few examples
of the questions he's been sent. Remember, the way we
learn is by asking. Go on, send him an e-mail.

Style dilemma? Who you gonna call?
Email AskTheGeek@TheChicGeek.co.uk

ASK THE GEEK

Hello Geek!

I am attending my mate's wedding next weekend but rather than fork out for a suit in a hurry, I thought I might just wear a nice shirt and trouser combo. Perhaps with a tie/dickie bow. Is there any chance you could help me in assembling an outfit? I was thinking maybe some dark grey slim trousers, but I'm not too sure about shirt colour. What do you think?! Thanks Geek! Si

Hey Si

How about a nice plain sky-blue shirt with a darker blue velvet bow-tie? These would be great with the grey trousers and would look tasteful yet stylish. I would also try a pair of navy patent shoes to complement the tie – perfect for a winter wedding and, with it being dark for longer, looks great under low lighting. The Geek

Hi There

I was wondering if you can help me, please. I want to buy a winter coat as a present for my boyfriend. I've been on three shopping trips but to no avail. He is a shortish, slim, yet well-built gent. Any suggestions on what style/brand might suit him? A smart coat preferably and the budget is open to anything really, once it's stylish. Any help you can give me would be massively appreciated. Kellie

Hi Kellie

Lucky boyfriend! You say he is shortish so I wouldn't go for a long coat as it usually swamps a bit and will make him look shorter. I suggest a peacoat shape – the double breasting will balance his top half and show his legs which will make him look taller. The Geek

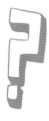

Hi Geek

I need a really sharp suit and I want something a bit different and trendy, but not wanting to break the bank. Any thoughts? Cheers, Mike

Hi Mike

On a budget I would go for something simple. Stick to a two-button single-breasted suit in grey or navy. Marks & Spencer have started to do slim-fitting suits in their Limited Collection; other places to try are Ben Sherman or Lambretta, who do very sharp Mod-style suits, which have become modern classics and Topman is really good for affordable yet slick tailoring. Remember though Mike, fit is everything, so try it on to make sure you look and feel comfortable in it. Hope this helps. The Geek

Dear *Chic* Geek

I'm looking at buying a tailored blazer/jacket, essentially for casual and smart use but something I can wear with lots of different things. My influences in style are those like George Lamb, Sauvage, etc. I wanted something quite sharp and slim but something that would stand out in terms of fabric. Can you give me any ideas before I head down to a tailor? Kind regards, Andrew

Hi Andrew

I know you didn't specify a colour but I immediately thought navy. You'll get the most wear out of a navy jacket; it looks so good with white and colour during the warmer months. Made from silk/cotton voile, the jacket would go with everything and the relaxed fabric will look great all season long. As for detailing, if you're having something made, Paul Smith puts distressed silk on his lapels and uses de-structured construction and fabric cut slim. Double-breasted can look good during the summer months but keep the fabric light as it could get hot and it looks best done up. The Geek

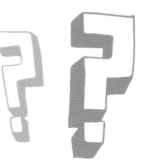

Hi Geek

What is your opinion about teaming a slimfit black Timothy Everest velvet suit with wine trim with a smartish shirt and Paul Smith burgundy velvet bow-tie? Should we really opt for the trad white dress shirt?   Thanks, Julia

Hi Julia

If this is for the groom, can't wait to hear what you are wearing!

This sounds good, just make sure everything is fitted and the whole look is really sharp and tight. Try different collar sizes with the bow-tie to see what you like best. Dress shirts are nice because they have detailing but a plain, good-quality white shirt would be fine – as I say, it's all about the collar size and proportion. May I suggest some wine- or brown-coloured patent shoes to finish the look? On a grooming note, keep it quite natural; there's a line between referencing a look and fancy dress. Hope this helps.   The Geek

Yo Geek

I've been invited for a day aboard a friend's boat, I'm not really sure what to wear as it's my first time. What would your advice be?   Thanks, Patrick

Hi Patrick

You can go two ways; technical or classic. Whichever one you choose, consider layering. It's usually a few degrees cooler near water, so when you get out there you want to have the option of adding or taking away. I would start with a T-shirt, then add a piece of knitwear – something rustic like an Aran or maybe a nice white and navy horizontal stripe sweater. You can take this off if you get too hot.

For the technical look, add a synthetic/waterproof jacket from somewhere like Zegna Sport or Prada Sport, or for more a classic style, try a double-breasted blazer. Add boat shoes for a non-slip option and you're good to go, sailor!   CG

Dear *Chic* Geek

My boyfriend sports the geek-chic look but often looks gangly and stupid because of his extreme height. (He's almost 7 foot tall.) Any advice for the giant-looking people of this world? Something that would look good on him and not make him look like he borrowed a kid's clothes? Brands? Stores? anything? Ha ha.   Thanks, Roxi

Hi Roxi

Extremes can be difficult, 7 foot is very tall but there's certainly nothing wrong with that. I would suggest sticking with classic pieces; if you try and go too trendy, it looks too young on somebody so tall. You say he does the geek-chic look so I presume he is quite slim. Designers often leave their trousers unfinished so they can be as long as you want, but you have the hassle and expense of alterations. I would stay away from tailored clothes as these are clothes you judge on their exact fit. I would go for shirts, T-shirts and knitwear, the type of items you can "tszuj" (roll up or push up) the arms a little, making it look more casual. The choice of items becomes smaller the taller you get. I would suggest, say for summer, rolling the trousers up above the ankles and wearing loafers with no socks – it's about styling what you've got. Buy simple clothes but style on the shoes and sunglasses. Or if you have the confidence to pull it off, the whole vintage/shrunken look can work. I bought a 1960s American DB jacket which is way too small on the arms but because it fits well on the body, it works and is different yet smart. So if one area fits well, you can go slightly different on another length. Good luck.

The Geek

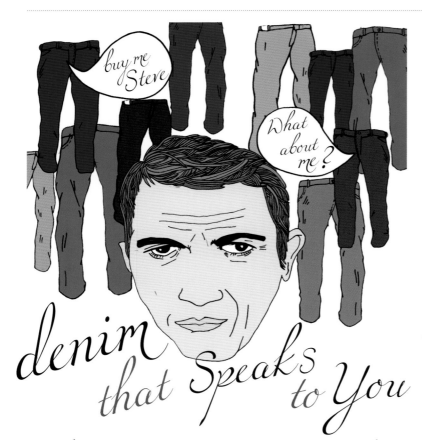

buy me Steve

What about me?

When buying jeans, you should always go with denim that speaks to you, you should listen to your instinct. Find jeans that make your butt look good and it always helps to shop with your girlfriend or significant other. Honesty is critical.

J Brand Denim Company's co-founder Jeff Rudes

denim that Speaks to You

Dear *Chic* Geek

I'm looking for a pair of jeans that will be flattering and versatile, but there are so many brands on the market. Can you tell me which colour and cut to go for?   Steve

Dear Steve

The perfect pair of jeans are the ones you love. An overdyed black wash is a great option that will take the working man from the office to the bar, dinner party or anywhere else he intends to go when his day at work is done. The tall, skinny guy should stick with the slim, straight leg, while slightly portly guys look good in a fuller bootleg with a dark wash. The shorter guy suits a bootcut as well, but a stovepipe straight leg is also flattering. The jean should not be too baggy from the thigh to the knee.   The Geek

Dear *Chic* Geek

What styles suit an average black guy? I am six feet tall and a 32-inch waist with 42-inch jacket or large shirt. What clothes would suit me best when I'm going out to a club, bar or just chilling?   Thanks, Andy

Hi Andy

I would go quite preppy. Black guys really suit that Kanye West, Andre 3000, slightly geeky-preppy look. Wear a nice shirt with a fitted, thin V-neck sweater to show off your body. Straight-leg jeans and fresh white trainers. Keep it all very clean and crisp.   The Geek

Dear Mr Geek

I am met with a dilemma of practicality versus presentability. Next year I plan to travel around Europe, however as a classical musician I would like to take smart clothing to allow me to perform in the various cities I visit. Ideally I would like to avoid using a suit carrier as over the distances planned it will inevitably become rather tiresome, particularly as I hope to go by motorcycle for part of the way. Is there any cunning trick of the trade for folding one's suit to avoid catastrophic crumpling and spoiling the shape, or is this completely unavoidable?   Yours sincerely, Fred Platt

Hi Fred

Sounds like quite a trip. Lose the suit carrier and take what is practical to enjoy the ride. There's no way to avoid some sort of creasing, but what you can do is put tissue paper or newspaper inside the suit to minimize wrinkles. Your suit will need pressing to look its best, so you have two options: take a travel iron/steamer or ask your hotel or local dry cleaner to press it for a small charge.

You often read about suits that don't crease and ways of packing to avoid creasing, but nothing looks better than a newly ironed item of clothing, especially when playing in front of an audience.   The Geek

Dear *Chic* Geek

I recently had a heated discussion about wearing flip-flops out to a bar. I think they look fine with a pair of shorts and a T-shirt, my mate thought otherwise, so I just wondered what your opinion was.   Thanks, Chris

Dear Chris

Are you an Australian by any chance? Flip-flops regardless of the brand seem too relaxed; they also make your feet look a little dirty. They shouldn't be worn away from the beach or pool and if you're in a bar at night in town, then never. I'm surprised they let you in! Try a pair of sandals or, better still, boat shoes are great with shorts, formal but not too formal, and extremely comfortable. Good luck.   The Geek

Hi Geek

I like to wear my clothes quite fitted and this time of year all my white T-shirts and shirts get those horrible yellow armpit stains which don't come out in a normal wash. Is there anything I can do?   Matt

Hi Matt

You're probably like the rest of us when it comes to washing our clothes – just shove it in the machine and hope for the best. But some things do need a little TLC, like armpit stains. We are told that prevention is better than cure, so the first thing to do is to try and minimize getting the stains in the first place. When you apply deodorant, make sure your armpits are completely dry first. Wait a couple of minutes before putting on your shirt or T-shirt to let the deodorant dry, as this is one of the main causes of yellow armpit stains. Avoid antiperspirants with aluminium zirconium tetrachlorohydrex gly as the active ingredient, which may contribute to the sweat stains.

Here are some more tips:

• Avoid heat. Hot water or heat from the dryer will set the stains. Rinse the item in cold water and allow it to air dry.

• Avoid bleach. If the shirt is white, you might be tempted to bleach the stain. Don't. Bleach will actually darken the stain because it reacts with the proteins in sweat.

• When you wash your white shirts, put some baking soda in with your laundry detergent. This will lessen the yellow underneath the armpits and helps keep the entire shirt white, rather than a yellowish faded colour over time. You can buy a whitening product that will whiten your clothes with every wash. Treat stubborn stains by rubbing the whitening powder directly onto the area with cold water and then washing – follow the individual instructions on the packaging.

• Dry natural fabrics in sunlight as this helps to break down the stain further.

• If the stain is yellow or green in colour and has a crunchy or crispy texture, it's due to perspiration. If the stain is white or clear with a greasy texture, this is down to the antiperspirant and should be treated as a grease stain. Hope this helps.   The Geek

Dear *Chic* Geek

I have been updating my wardrobe over the last six months and tried on a pair of Pointer Cyril Desert Boots, but I really can't decide which colour out of charcoal, dark brown or tan to purchase. I plan to mostly wear them with straight indigo jeans and will also be buying a pair of Dr Denim chinos afterward in either khaki, navy or grey. I also plan to buy a tweed jacket or creased-type blazer to wear with this look. What colour do you think would go best with the type of clothes I am describing and generally would be versatile? It is unusual to see shoes in the grey colour, I think, but I'm sure the light brown would work better.

Many thanks, Jason

Hi Jason

You sound like you've got a great wardrobe going on there. I don't happen to like the suede/leather contrast ones, regardless of colour, but I quite like the mahogany ones, which I think will age nicely. I would have said dark brown, as I've been wearing Clark's Camden Lock in dark brown all autumn and they are great and go with everything particularly dark blue jeans. Suede seems to suit dark brown rather than other colours. The ChicGeek

Hi *Chic* Geek

I have to wear smart leather shoes to work but find most pairs extremely uncomfortable by the end of the day. Is there anything you can recommend? Many thanks, Joe

Hi Joe

It's strange how some shoes never get more comfortable through wear and eventually you just give up on them. Good news. Footwear brand Rockport has launched a new range of shoes called DresSport, a shoe that combines the aesthetic of a smart shoe with the comfort technology of trainers (sneakers). To prove just how comfortable these shoes are, two teams competed in the Dublin and New York marathons wearing them. Both teams completed the race.

The Geek

Dear Geek

There is nothing I like better than to retreat to the countryside and on a Saturday night tour several countryside pubs drinking real ale and getting drunk with the lads. What do you recommend I wear, bearing in mind most of the places I frequent have well-spoken clientèle and matching bar staff, drive Chelsea tractors with white and yellow name tags and have several acres of back garden. I have tried the Superdry T-shirt and light denim jeans with trainers but it doesn't seem to bode well. On the other hand, I really don't fancy tweed so stuck between the two... Look forward to hearing your thorough recommendations.

Sincerely yours, Edward J Lancaster Esq.

Hi Edward

The Superdry T-shirt and light denims with trainers is more Walkabout theme bar than White Hart country pub. You should look casual but English casual. This fitted T-shirt and frayed jean look has spread across the globe quicker then swine flu and to be honest is now quite dated. Let's start with the shoes, go for a traditional brown English brogue. Grenson are great and really affordable (www.grenson. co.uk). Add a fitted, straight-leg jean in a nice indigo or rich blue, then a cashmere or merino wool knitted V-neck. Wear over a plain T-shirt and finish with a nice Barbour waxed jacket. They are doing some really cool styles at the moment and the quality for the price is amazing. Add a smile and the locals are going to love you.

The Geek

Hi *Chic* Geek

I bought a great cashmere jacket from the Nick Hart for Aquascutum range last year, but it's started to bobble badly on the bottoms of the arms and beginning to look a bit shabby. What's the best way to get rid of the bobbles?

Cheers, Jon

Hello Jon

Wow, nice jacket! The best way to get rid of the bobbles is with a battery-operated clothes shaver. You simply move it over the problem areas and the bobbles are collected in the machine. Hope this helps. Best wishes, The Geek

Hey *Chic* Geek

I dearly love my beige chinos that I've recently bought but what would you suggest would be the best overall look to go with them?   Nishan

Hi Nishan

The beige chino was, until recently, associated with preppies and Sloanes so the best thing to do is to wear them with irony and subvert the look. Team with tassel loafers and if the trousers are slightly tapered, you could roll them up above the ankle. As for the top half, I would wear a crisp monogrammed polo-shirt or a plain round-neck T-shirt in grey or navy. Keep the look clean, cool preppy. Liberty of London have some great polo shirts covered in flies or you could just go for a classic from Ralph Lauren or Lacoste in white. As for T-shirts, I think the best are from Sunspel.

Hope this helps. CG

Hi CG

I have recently purchased some dark red loafers and was wondering what colour sock would best suit? Or perhaps pattern?   Thanks, Si

Hi Si,

I would go for berry colours in any pattern. I really like houndstooth or herringbone at the moment. I saw a stunning pair of deep purple Richard James' cashmere socks – he does the best patterns and colours. The cashmere ones are expensive but the wool ones are cheaper and still in beautiful colours.   The Chic Geek

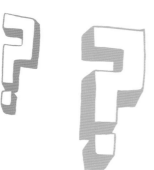

Hey Geek

I usually use hair wax to style my hair but in the summer I've found in the heat and sun it just doesn't last or hold, Can you recommend anything that will do the job better?

Cheers, Jim

Hi Jim

I've recently had the same problem. The heat seems to make the wax disappear. I was recommended Label m matt paste, which has more hold without making your hair hard or too rigid. It works pretty well and also contains a thing called the Enviroshield Complex, which shields against UV rays too, which is good for your hair. Hope this helps.

The Geek

Hi Geek

I've been trying to grow my sideburns but they are a bit wispy. Is there anything I do to thicken them up a bit?

Cheers, Matt

Hi Matt

Unfortunately there is nothing you can do except shave them off. It is better to have no sideburns then little tufts of bum fluff on either side of your face. Facial hair is a difficult one, you can either do it or you can't. The hair on some men's faces grows better in different areas, but take some consolation from the fact that a lack of sideburns will leave you looking younger.   The Geek

Hello CG

I've got very fair skin so I burn easily in the sun. I've been using high factor creams as recommended but they seem to give me spots. What can I do?   Martin

Dear Martin

This is a problem with high-factor creams as they are very thick and combined with perspiring more in the sun can cause spots. I would recommend opting for a lower factor SPF, say a 15 SPF or 20 SPF, but reapplying more often. If you are particularly fair, limit your skin exposure anyway especially in the middle of the day.   Best, The Chic Geek

RAGLAN SLEEVE **R**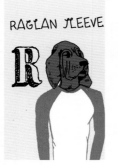

P PORK PIE HAT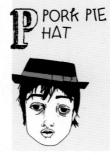

G GAUNTLET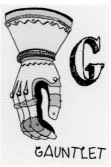

B BEAVER-LAMB FUR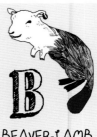

JERSEY **J** 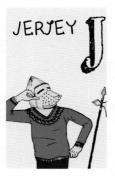 FAIRISLE

F 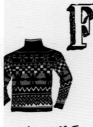 FAIRISLE

E ERMINE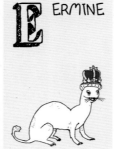

H HIGHRISE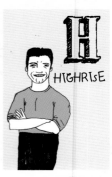

A 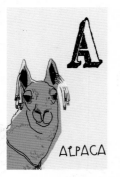 ALPACA

KARAKUL **K**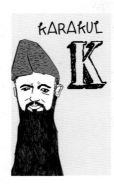

MADRAS CHECK **M**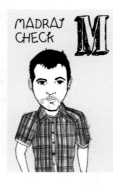

OXFORD BAGS **O**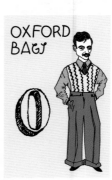

LAPEL **L**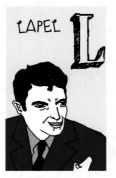

D DEALER BOOT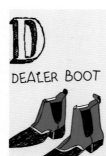

C CRAVAT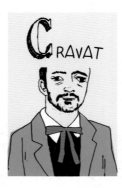

N NEHRU JACKET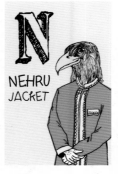

Geekipedia

If you're unsure of something **The Chic Geek** has previously said or would simply like to know more regarding the origins of a particular word or menswear term, then here is the Geekipedia – The Chic Geek's own Wikipedia of style terms.

A glossary of fashion terminology for those who want to know their alpaca from their Zoot suit, the Geekipedia fills in the blanks. Here you can find out which earl the cardigan is named after and why ponyskin isn't really made out of ponies – just straight-talking explanations of anything to do with what a man wears.

GEEKIPEDIA

Alpaca – *al-pak-a* Cloth made from the long silken wool of the Peruvian llama, normally used to make coats. The texture is fluffy, almost teddybear-like.

Angora – *an-gora* The extremely soft and warm hair of the Angora rabbit. Your mum probably had a sweater made from this in the 1980s with cats or something just as tacky or grotesque on the front.

Aran A style of sweater that takes its name from the Aran Islands off the west coast of Ireland. It has prominent cable patterns on the chest and is often cream-coloured. The sweaters are distinguished by the use of complex textured stitch patterns, several of which are combined in the creation of a single garment. It was primarily the wives of island fishermen who knitted them. Some stitch patterns have a traditional interpretation, often of religious significance. The honeycomb is a symbol of the hard-working bee; the cable, an integral part of the fisherman's daily life, is said to be a wish for safety and good luck when fishing; the diamonds a wish for success, wealth and treasure while the basket stitch represents the fisherman's basket, a hope for a plentiful catch.

Astrakhan – *as-tra-kan* The pelts of very young or foetal lambs; the fur is very tight and curly. Often used in hats and collars on coats. Hamid Karzai, President of Afghanistan, is always seen wearing a Karakul hat made from astrakhan or "Persian lamb" as it is sometimes called.

Balmacaan A looser-fitting, single-breasted coat which has a raglan sleeve, usually a raincoat. Designed in Scotland, the idea being that fewer seams would lower the risk of water creeping in.

Barathea – *bara-thea* Worsted fabric with twill hopsack weave; silk or silk-and-worsted fabric with lightly ribbed or pebbled weave. Usually used for dress clothes, blazers and uniforms.

Batik The art of decorating cloth using wax and dye. It has been practised for centuries and in Java, Indonesia, batik is part of an ancient tradition. The word "batik" originates from the Javanese *tik* and means "to dot".

Beaver-lamb Fur Lambskin sheared to look like beaver.

Beret – *ber-ray* A round, flat cap usually made of wool and traditionally associated with French peasants or elite military units.

Bespoke Derives from the word "bespeak", meaning "to ask for" and originates from London's Savile Row, where a customer would "bespeak" a measure of cloth. The bespoke bolt of cloth was not available to any other client until the entire suit had been cut, assembled and sewn. Bespoke is often confused with "made to measure" but is not simply a process of tailoring measurements; it allows the wearer to choose materials, colours and any details they specifically request and it is also entirely hand-sewn. This is the ultimate in male dressing, the haute couture of menswear.

Bias – *bye-ass* The term for when the fabric is cut diagonally across the grain of the weave.

Binding This is the tape sewn into the inside of the bottom of your trousers, without which the constant rubbing on your shoes might cause unsightly fraying.

Bird's Eye A fabric woven with a pattern of small diamonds, each having a dot in the centre.

Black Tie This term has changed somewhat. There was once a time when we were afraid to be underdressed and now the reverse is true. Generally "black tie" means a dinner jacket (tuxedo). Anything else you team with the jacket is up to your personality and individuality, but never trainers (sneakers), please.

Blazer Usually brightly coloured and sporting metal buttons, the blazer originated in the 1860s as a short jacket with patch pockets worn for tennis and cricket. It has had something of a bad image, thanks to Alan Partridge and his "sports casual" look.

Boat Shoe Sometimes called deck shoes or topsiders, boat shoes were invented by Paul Sperry in 1935 and said to be inspired by Sperry's cocker spaniel, Prince, running across the ice on a winter's day in Connecticut. Noticing the tiny cracks and cuts going in all directions on Prince's paws, Sperry developed a patent called "razor-siping" on the soles, which provided a non-slip surface.

Boater – *bow-ter* A hard straw hat, usually seen on toffs when near water.

Bouclé – *boo-clay* A curled effect on the surface of a cloth producing small loops of thread; think the material in your granny's classic Chanel jacket.

Bow-tie The bow-tie originated among Croatian mercenaries during the Prussian wars of the seventeenth century. It consists of a ribbon of fabric tied around the collar in a symmetrical manner such that the two opposite ends form loops. Today, there is something slightly eccentric (in a good way) associated with wearing bow ties away from the traditional realms of black tie. The Chic Geek calls it "*Antique Roadshow* chic".

Bowler Hat   A stiff, felted hat with a round-ish brim named after the London hatmakers Thomas and William Bowler, who first made it in 1849. Called a "derby" in America.

Breeches   Trousers that come to the knee. The eighteenth-century equivalent of cycling shorts, they are also called "breeks" or "knickerbockers". You can still pick up a pair in James Purdey and Sons in Mayfair for those days spent on the grouse moor.

Brim   The rim of a hat.

Brocade – *brok-caid*   This is a richly decorated fabric, usually silk woven with gold or silver thread. Comes from the Italian *broccato*, meaning "embossed cloth".

Brogue – *b-rogue*   A stout shoe with a form of decorative punching of the upper leather of shoes. The word comes from the Scottish or Irish Gaelic word *brog*, meaning "shoe". They are known as "wingtips" in America because the design on the upper toe looks like a bird's outspread wings.

Camelhair   The soft hair from the underside of the camel, usually in a biscuity brown colour.

Cardigan   A knitted woollen jacket fastened with buttons or a zip. The cardigan was named after James Thomas Brudenell, 7th Earl of Cardigan

and a British military commander, following his service in the Crimean War (1797–1868).

Cashmere – *kash-mer*   The soft downy undercoat of the cashmere goat. The word "cashmere" derives from an archaic spelling of Kashmir, which borders India and Pakistan. The majority of today's cashmere wool comes from China.

Centre Vent   This is the slit in the middle of a jacket designed to allow the jacket to sit easily when the wearer is sitting astride a horse.

Chambray   A linen-finished gingham with a white weft and a coloured warp.

Chamois – *sham-wa*   A soft leather made from the goat-like antelope inhabiting mountains in southern and central Europe. Used to make gloves.

Chelsea Boot   An ankle-high leather boot with an elasticated side insert that allows the boot to be easily taken on and off. Associated with the 1960s and those groovy males strutting down Carnaby Street. Also know as "dealer boots".

Chesterfield   The Chesterfield coat is a long, tailored overcoat. It can be single- or double-breasted and has been popular in a wide variety of fabrics, typically heavier-weight tweeds, and in charcoal and navy. It often has a velvet collar. Named after the style of coat worn by the Earl of Chesterfield during the eighteenth century, it is often confused with a Crombie.

Cheviot Tweed – *che-vi-ot*   A tweed made from the hardy breed of short-woolen sheep reared on the range of rolling hills straddling the

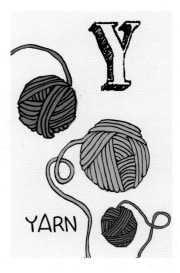

YARN

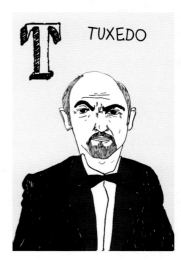

TUXEDO

England/Scotland border between Northumberland and the Scottish Borders called the Cheviot Hills. It has become a general title covering many kinds of rough tweed.

Chinos In 1848, Sir Harry Lumsden, commanding officer of a British regiment in India, had the idea to dye his men's white uniform with a mixture of coffee, curry powder and mulberry juice to disguise the inevitable dirt. The Indians called this new colour "khaki". The name chino comes from the fact that these trousers were originally made in China – *chino* is the Spanish term for Chinese.

Co-respondents Usually a two-tone brogue in black and white or brown and white. The story goes that an unusually patterned or coloured pair of men's shoes was left outside the hotel room in which adultery was taking place, ostensibly to be cleaned, but in fact as a signal that adultery was taking place within. The name is derived from legal parlance wherein the co-respondent is the third party or lover in the ensuing divorce case.

Codpiece A codpiece – from Middle English cod, "scrotum" – is a covering flap or pouch that attaches to the front of the crotch of men's trousers and usually accentuates the genital area.

Cordovan Leather Fine leather from horses, named after Cordoba, Spain.

Corduroy – *kor-do-roy* Corduroy is a ribbed cotton velvet which forms distinctive cord-like shapes in the fabric. The word comes from *Corde du Roi*, which is roughly translated from the French as the "cloth/cord of the King". It is difficult to imagine a French

king wearing anything as hardwearing and outdoorsy as corduroy but it is said that his servants wore the fabric while hunting. Believed to have first been produced in Manchester, England, some Germans still call it "Manchester". The width of the cord is commonly referred to as the size of the "wale". The lower the wale number, the thicker the width of the cord.

Cossack Hat – *kos-ak* A brimless hat of fur or similar material. This is the typical fur hat seen on Soviet soldiers.

Cotton Long, soft hairs covering the seed of the cotton plant (*Gossypium*). The English name began to be used in the thirteenth and fourteenth centuries and derives from the Arabic *qutun*. Cotton is a pesticide-intensive crop using about 25 per cent of the world's insecticides and 10 per cent of the world's pesticides so it is important to purchase organic cotton when available.

Cravat – *krav-at* A neck cloth chiefly worn by men. It was introduced in 1636 from the Cravates, or Croatians. In the reign of France's Louis XIII Croatian mercenaries were enlisted into a regiment supporting the King and Cardinal Richelieu. The traditional Croat military kit aroused Parisian curiosity about the unusual scarves distinctively knotted around the Croatians' necks. It was the forerunner of today's necktie and bow-tie.

Crease Smartens a pair of trousers and emphasizes the line of the trousers. Never let your mother iron them into your jeans!

Crewneck The round, close-fitting, high-neck jersey worn by crews on rowing teams.

Crombie – *krom-bee* A Crombie is a man's long woollen overcoat, usually made in a dark colour with a contrasting brightly coloured lining with a concealed packet button fastening. The name of J&J Crombie Limited, a Scottish firm of clothmakers, once designated the type of overcoat, jacket, etc., made by them.

Crown The top part of a hat.

Cufflink A pair of decorative fasteners or one button-like object attached to a pivoting bar used for fastening a double-cuff shirt. Cufflinks come in many guises; the best solution is to keep them simple – no clever slogans or joke cufflinks; classic gold ovals are the best. Often worn by stockbrokers, cufflinks haven't been fashionable for a while and feel a little too dated.

Cummerbund – *kum-ar-bund* A waist-belt or a sash. The name comes from the Urdu and Persian *kamar-band*, from *kamar* "waist, loins" and *bandi* "band" in the seventeenth century.

Dart A tapering fold sewn onto the reverse of material in order to shape the cloth to the body's contours.

Dealer Boot *see* Chelsea boot.

Deerstalker A cap with side flaps that can be tied onto the top. It is the type of hat that Sherlock Holmes is usually depicted wearing.

Denim Twilled cotton fabric used for overalls and jeans. The word comes from the name of a sturdy fabric called serge, originally made in Nîmes, France. First called *serge de Nîmes*, the name was quickly shortened to "denim".

Derby The American term for a Bowler hat.

Dinner Jacket An English term for what is known as a tuxedo in the USA and a smoking jacket in Germany.

Doeskin A woollen cloth made to look like a doe's skin by felting. It has a smooth, velvety finish.

Dogtooth Check *See* Houndstooth Check.

Donegal Tweed An Irish tweed originally woven in County Donegal, which has a rough, knobbly surface. It is often woven with dark and light flecks and the pattern is generally called "pepper and salt". This is a very stylish tweed to wear as a single-breasted suit during the autumn and winter months.

Dress Shirt A shirt worn with tails or a tuxedo, usually with a wing or turndown collar.

Drill A stout twilled linen or cotton cloth used for shirts and shorts.

Ermine The stoat's winter coat – white fur dotted with black tail tips used on the ceremonial robes worn by kings and queens.

Fairisle A type of design used in knitwear and named after a Shetland island. History has it that a sixteenth-century Spanish Armada galleon was wrecked and the sailors rescued from the vessel wore garments bearing Moorish designs, which the Shetland islanders copied. Fairisle knitwear is hand-knitted wool with horizontal, coloured bands of naive or folky patterns and designs.

Felt A fabric formed without weaving, using the natural tendency of the fibres of wool or rabbit fur to interface and cling together into a mat-like texture. Felt is actually the oldest fabric known to humankind.

Fishtail The rear part of trousers cut specifically for braces (suspenders). The back panel is divided and pulled upward so that the waistcoat does not ride up into the waistband.

Fitch The pelt of the European polecat, used for coats and jackets and in trimmings.

Foulard The first meaning is a thin, flexible silk or silk and cotton material used for ties and handkerchiefs. It can also denote the actual scarves or handkerchiefs made from this fabric. The word comes from the French for a silk handkerchief.

Frog Pocket A form of cross pocket in the trousers with the seam end opened vertically a few inches so that it is easier to get your hand in.

Gaberdine A closely woven twill fabric made of cotton or wool. The fabric is smooth on one side and has a diagonally ribbed surface on the other. This breathable, weatherproof and tearproof fabric was developed by Thomas Burberry, first introduced in 1880 and patented in 1888.

Gauntlet A long glove covering the wrist, typically worn when driving.

Ghillie (or Gillie) Collar Named after a Highland chief's attendant. This is when a jacket can be fastened all the way up to the neck, like a coat, keeping the Scottish weather out.

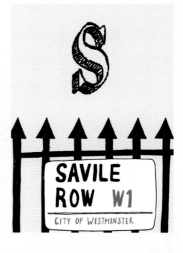

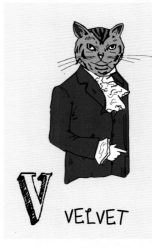

VELVET

Guernsey A close-fitting knitted upper garment, worn by sailors or fishermen.

Harris Tweed A hefty tweed hand-woven by islanders on the Isles of Harris, Lewis, Uist and Barra in the Outer Hebrides of Scotland, using local wool. As the Industrial Revolution reached Scotland, the mainland turned to mechanization but the Outer Islands retained their traditional processes. Every length of cloth produced is stamped with the official Orb symbol, trademarked by the Harris Tweed Association in 1909, when Harris Tweed was defined as "hand-spun, hand-woven and dyed by the crofters and cottars in the Outer Hebrides". The Harris Tweed Authority took over from the Harris Tweed Association in 1993 by Act of Parliament. Thus the definition of Harris Tweed became statutory and forever tied the cloth to the Islands. Harris Tweed means a tweed which has been handwoven by the islanders at their homes in the Outer Hebrides, finished in the islands of Harris, Lewis, North Uist, Benbecula, South Uist and Barra and their several purtenances (The Outer Hebrides) and made from pure virgin wool, dyed and spun in the Outer Hebrides.

Henley A collarless men's casualwear pullover shirt, characterized by a 10-15 cm (4–6 inch) long placket beneath the round neckline, usually having two or five buttons. It resembles a collarless polo shirt. Named because this particular style of shirt was the traditional uniform of rowers in the English town of Henley-on-Thames.

High Rise Trousers that come over your stomach; think "early days" Simon Cowell.

Homburg A semi-formal hat with a crease and no dents.

Hopsack A weave giving the cloth an appearance of minute squares.

Houndstooth Check A textile pattern of broken checks, often seen in black and white.

Hulden Check This is British label Aquascutum's signature check of beige and navy squares.

Intarsia Term used for a pattern inlaid into another.

Jersey – *jur-zi* Has two meanings: the Channel Island of Jersey was famous for its knitting trade in medieval times and the name refers to what today we would also call a sweater; a close-fitting, wool or cotton pullover. Jersey is also a soft, slightly elastic knit cloth made from wool, cotton or silk. The name derives from Jersey, the largest of the Channel Islands, where the material was first produced.

Kaftan Traditionally a man's cotton or silk cloak buttoned down the front, with full sleeves reaching to the ankles and worn with a sash. Today, the kaftan has come to mean a long, loose shirt-type garment with loose sleeves worn in the summer months.

Karakul – *kar-a-kool* A hat named after an Asiatic breed of sheep using the fur of very young lambs, also called astrakhan or Persian lamb. The hat is peaked with a rounded or flattened crown that lies flat when taken off.

Karung Another word for snakeskin.

Khakis *see* Chinos.

Knickerbockers Short, loose trousers gathered in at or just below the knees, as those worn by the Dutch settlers of New York.

Lapel – *la-pel* A part of the coat folded back, which continues on from the collar. There are three basic forms of lapel: notched, peaked and shawl. Notched are your common everyday lapels found on suits. Peaked lapels are more formal and nearly always used on double-breasted jackets or coats, with the point at the shoulders. Shawl is a rounded lapel without points usually found on dinner jackets.

Lawn Originally a linen material made in Laon, France, today it is mostly cotton and known for its semi-transparency.

Linen A textile made from the fibres of the flax plant, linen is valued for its coolness during warmer months.

Long Johns Underpants with long legs. The name is derived from the old boxing gear worn by John L Sullivan, who was a boxer in the late 1880s. They were sent out to soldiers during the First World War.

Lovat – *luv-at* Lovat is a heather mixture colour made of a blend of soft blues, greens and a little brown, usually found in tweed or woollen cloth.

Lurex Brand name for a type of yarn with a metallic appearance. The twine is most commonly a synthetic fibre onto which an aluminium layer has been vaporized. Lurex may also refer to cloth created with the yarn.

Mackintosh A form of waterproof raincoat, first sold in 1823 and made out of rubberized fabric. The Mackintosh is named after its Scottish inventor Charles Macintosh. The distinctive smell is like Marmite: you either love it or hate it.

Made-to-Measure This is the construction of an item of clothing, usually to suit your exact measurements. Made-to-measure manufacturers use both machine- and hand-sewing. Made-to-measure also requires fewer fittings than bespoke, resulting in a shorter wait between customer measurement and the final garment delivery.

Madras Check A fabric made of patches of plaid fabric, it is pure cotton fabric woven in the city of Madras, India. Known for its bleeding qualities and softness, making it ideal wear for summer, it is usually brightly coloured.

Maillot – *my-yo* A close-fitting knitted shirt (also a woman's swimsuit).

Marl A mottled yarn or fabric, classically seen in grey.

Matelot – *mat-lo* A stripy, blue and white sailor's jersey made famous by Jean Paul Gaultier. The male torso on the bottle of Gaultier's classic fragrance wears a matelot.

Melton – *mel-ton* A strong cloth for overcoats. It takes its name from Melton Mowbray in Northamptonshire, where it first came into general use.

Mercerize – *mur-cer-rise* To treat cotton so as to make it appear like silk. The process was devised in 1844 by John Mercer of Great Harwood,

Lancashire, England, who treated cotton fibres with sodium hydroxide to make them stronger and more absorbent for dyeing.

Merino Wool – *ma-re-no* Wool grown by the breed of Merino sheep. Superfine Merinos are regarded as having the finest and softest wool of any sheep. The majority of the wool comes from Australia.

Milan Collar Rather than a single button at the top, the Milan collar has two smaller buttons to fasten the collar.

Miniver – *min-i-ver* The soft underbelly of the grey squirrel.

Mohair The long, white, silken hair of the Angora goat.

Morning Suit Consists of a black or grey tailcoat, plus a waistcoat (often in a pale colour), striped or checked trousers with no turn-ups (cuffs) and a black or grey top hat. Despite its name, morning dress may be worn to afternoon social events before five o'clock, but not to events beginning after seven o'clock in the evening. This is the type of dress most associated with weddings and Royal Ascot.

Nehru Jacket – *ner-ru* A hip-length tailored coat with a stand-up or "mandarin" collar, no lapels and modelled on the South Asian *achkan* or *sherwani*, an apparel worn by Jawaharlal Nehru, the prime minister of India from 1947 to 1964.

Norfolk Jacket First worn on the estates of the Duke of Norfolk, this is a tweed jacket with three or four buttons, a belt, pleats for ease of movement and large pockets.

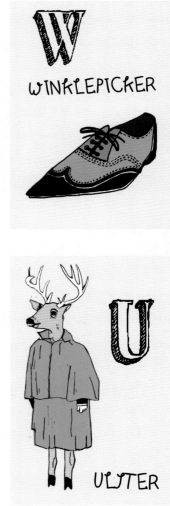

W

WINKLEPICKER

U

ULSTER

Notch – *noch* The cutout where your lapel meets the collar on your suit jacket.

Nylon This term describes the generic family of synthetic polymers known generically as polyamides and first produced on 28 February 1935 by Wallace Carothers at DuPont. It was one of the first manmade fibres. How nylon got its name is unclear, but one version from Dupont suggests they wanted to name it "No-Run" as it didn't unravel easily, but modified it to avoid making such an unjustified claim and to make the word sound better. Others say the name comes from the amalgamation of New York (NY) and London (LON), the places where it was first developed and launched.

Organza A thin, stiff, transparent dress fabric made of silk or a synthetic yarn.

Oxford Bags Loose-fitting, very wide and baggy trousers favoured by members of the University of Oxford during the beginning of the twentieth century. Always synonymous with the 1920s and 1930s.

Oxford Shirt This is a shirt with a button-down collar. It originally started on the polo field in England when players fastened the collars to the shirt with buttons to stop them flapping in their faces while playing. John Brooks of Brooks Brothers saw this and took the idea back to New York, adding the detail onto the shirt in 1896 and the classic American staple was born.

P.O.A. – Price On Application. This is usually reserved for a special piece that has to be ordered as a one-off from the designer or brand at the beginning of the season.

Paisley Vibrant pattern typified by a comma or teardrop shape. Persian in origin, paisley print derives its name from the town of Paisley in central Scotland. The brightly coloured, almost psychedelic patterning makes paisley associated with the 1960s. Christopher Bailey has experimented with paisley at Burberry and Liberty, which has some great paisley-style prints called Mark and Bourton in its archives.

Parka A warm, hip-length weatherproof coat with a fur-trimmed hood, originally worn by the Inuit. Originally made from caribou or seal, it was invented by the Caribou Inuit of the Arctic region, who needed clothing that would protect them from wind chill and wet while hunting and kayaking. The word "parka" is of Aleut origin.

Patent Leather Leather with a very shiny, glossy finish. Modern patent leather usually has a plastic finish. Good black patent should resemble crude oil. Once worn only with evening dress, patent shoes have proved very popular with any kind of trouser, day or night.

Peacoat This outer coat, generally of a navy-coloured heavy wool, was originally worn by sailors of European navies. Peacoats are characterized by broad lapels, double-breasted fronts, often large wooden or metal buttons and vertical or slash pockets. A "bridge coat" is a peacoat that extends to the thighs and is a uniform exclusively for officers and chief petty officers. The "reefer" is for officers only and is identical to the basic design but usually has gold buttons and epaulettes. The peacoat was named after the warm woollen fabric called *pij* that the Dutch used to make their sailor's jackets.

Penny Loafer A traditional slip-on with a strip of leather covering the top of the tongue and a "penny slot" design in the centre.

Pepper and Salt *see* Donegal Tweed.

Piqué – *pe-kay* A stiff corded cotton fabric mostly seen on the collars of polo shirts.

Placket A common term in menswear, this is the strip of fabric at the centre-front of a button-front shirt. If something is described as having a concealed placket, this means the buttons are covered by fabric so you don't see them.

Plaid – *plad* Americans tend to call check patterns "plaids" and this is becoming more common in the UK too. It also means the long, usually tartan, piece of cloth worn over the shoulder as part of Highland dress.

Pleats A fold or crease sewn or pressed into cloth that gathers a wider piece of fabric into a narrower area. Mostly seen on the front of old men's trousers, pleats can look very chic when exaggerated.

Plus-fours Very Bertie Wooster on the golf course. Derived from knickerbockers but 10 cm (4 inches) longer, hence the "plus four" so they overhang the fastening.

Ponyskin This is actually cowhide with the hair left on one side. It is not made from ponies or horses.

Poplin A plain-weave cotton fabric with slightly pronounced ribs running across it, poplin consists of a silk warp with a weft of worsted yarn. Shirts made from this fabric are easier to iron.

Porkpie Hat This hat gets its name from a resemblance to an English pork pie. The crown is flat with a rim like the crust found on the pie. Typically made of felt.

Prince of Wales Check The term is commonly applied to almost any Glen Urquhart check, particularly in black and white as often favoured by the Duke of Windsor. The understanding is that the original Prince of Wales check was designed by Edward VII for country and shooting use in Scotland and is a very large check with a repeat of 23 cm (9 inches) in bold red or brown on a cream ground with a grey over check. Commonly seen in a light suit fabric, it is a fine check overlaid with a colour check and where the fine checks cross over they bleed into a houndstooth-type patterned square. It had a moment in the late 1980s when every window cleaner made good was seen sporting a double-breasted Prince of Wales grey suit, but this is such a beautiful check that it is returning in a big way.

PTU Permanent Turn-Up (cuff).

Pullover This is pretty much is what it says it is: a knitted garment pulled over the head with no opening at the front.

Pyjama The word "pyjama" traces its etymological origin to the Persian word *payjama*, meaning "leg garment". However, it was first incorporated into English from the Hindustani language. During the seventeenth century, British men wore pyjamas as casual attire while relaxing until they became outmoded. They soon gained ground in the West during the colonial era and became popular as sleepwear, with designs inspired from similar traditional Indian and Persian garments. In India, pyjamas comprised important items of clothing for both women and Sikh men. It's about the piping, the pockets and the relaxed neck.

Raglan Sleeve A raglan sleeve runs all the way up the collar of a coat rather than attaching to the body at the shoulder, as is normal in shirts or suit jackets. It allows more movement and is therefore more sporting. Named after Lord Raglan because of the coat he wore while commanding his troops in the Crimea during the 1850s.

Rand A leather strip attached to the back of a shoe sole to level it before the heel is put on.

Romper An all-in-one shirt and short combination. Brings to mind people in skates but has found prominence in London's trendier circles.

RTW – Ready to Wear. Also known as "off-the-peg", meaning clothes that are completely finished when you buy them.

Sack Suit The Sack suit is an American term for a business suit and is defined as being a three-to-two blazer without darts and a single vent. Pioneered by classic American brand Brooks Brothers and seen on every young executive in the *Mad Men* television series.

Saffiano Leather This is the heavily grained or cross-hatched, waterproof and durable leather used by the Italian luxury goods houses of Prada and Salvatore Ferragamo.

Satin A closely woven, smooth, light-reflecting silk fabric of fairly heavy weight.

Savile Row Named after Lady Dorothy Savile, wife of the 3rd Earl of Burlington, Savile Row is a street in Mayfair, London, that is synonymous with bespoke men's tailoring. The term "Savile Row" describes any clothing made on or around the street by the multitude of tailoring houses. This is men's clothing at its finest, in both quality and history.

Scyes Armholes are also known as "scyes", which is a cutter's term. The majority of ready-made suits have large scyes, primarily to ensure the jacket fits most people.

Sea Island Cotton This is cotton from the Caribbean, the favourable conditions make the fibre longer and thus superfine and of high quality.

Seersucker A cotton fabric woven in such a way that some threads bunch together, giving the fabric a wrinkled appearance in places. Traditionally associated with the summer months, the word came into English from Hindi, which originates from the Persian words *shir o shakar*, meaning "milk and sugar", probably from the resemblance of its smooth and rough stripes to the smooth surface of milk and bumpy texture of sugar. The wrinkled appearance actually causes the fabric to be held away from the skin when worn, facilitating improved heat dissipation and air circulation.

Serge A heavy twill cotton with a fairly rough texture.

Shagreen This is leather commonly made from the skins of sharks and rays. The word derives from the French *chagrin*, meaning anxiety, annoyance – a reference to the rasping surface of the leather. Extremely hardwearing and usually seen in an *eau de nil* green colour with lighter, almost white circular markings, it is associated with the Art Deco era of the 1930s; even the wallpaper in the suites of Claridge's hotel in London is in the shagreen colour and pattern.

Shawl Collar A type of lapel usually found on dinner jackets, which is rounded with no points or strong angles.

Silk The best-known type of silk is obtained from cocoons made by the larvae of the mulberry silkworm, *Bombyx mori*. A fibre formed by the hardening of a liquid emitted from spinning-glands.

Snood A tubular neck protector or scarf. The garment can be worn either pulled down around the neck like a scarf or pulled up over the hair and lower face like a hood. The word is first recorded in Olde English from around 725.

Storm Collar A deep, often tabbed, collar that covers the neck fully when turned up.

Suede The inside or flesh side of leather that has been brushed or buffed into a velvety finish. Most often found in shoes and coats.

Tam o'Shanter A Scottish beret named after a character in a poem written by Robert Burns in 1790 and now traditionally worn by Rastafarians to hold their dreadlocks.

Tana Lawn Liberty of London made famous their tana lawn, which began manufacture in the 1920s. It is named after Lake Tana in Sudan, where the raw cotton was grown.

Tartan A pattern consisting of criss-crossed horizontal and vertical bands in multiple colours. Tartans originated in woven cloth but are now used in many other materials. Particularly associated with Scottish clans and regiments, the most famous tartan patterns are Black Watch and Royal Stewart. Scottish kilts almost always have tartan patterns.

Tattersall – *tat-ter-sol* A windowpane-type check mostly commonly found on shirts worn by farmers and woven in cotton, especially flannel. The pattern features thin dark lines forming squares on a light background.

Terry Towelling Terrycloth, terry cloth, terry towelling, terry or simply towelling is a fabric with loops that can absorb large amounts of water. Popular in the 1970s, it is very Riviera chic!

Tonic A fabric that changes colour as it moves;, very popular with suiting in the 1960s and 1970s.

Toscana Shearling A variety of lambskin usually characterized by a suede finish on the exterior and long fur (about 2.5 cm / 1 inch) on the interior of the pelt.

Trilby A soft felt hat with a deeply creased crown and snap-brim. Named after the George du Maurier novel *Trilby* (1894) because one was worn in the original London production.

Trouser Break This is the break where the trouser meets the shoe. The proper length for trousers is a "full break" or slight break in the crease. A full break means trousers are hemmed to reach the top of the heel of a standard dress shoe, naturally breaking over the front of the shoe.

Trouser Rise How much the trousers will rise up your legs when you sit down, generally anything from 5-10 cm (2–4 inches).

Tszuj - *zhuj* A fashion word which means to tweak your outfit, be it rolling up the sleeves or turning up your jeans.

Tuxedo American term for a dinner jacket named after the Tuxedo Park Club in New York in 1886 after one of the members was seen wearing a short smoking jacket made for him by Henry Poole & Co. in London and soon the informal dinner jacket caught on.

Tweed The name comes from a mistake. According to the Duke of Windsor, a clerk in around 1830 wrote "tweed" instead of "tweels", which meant twills to the Scots. "Scottish tweeds" were ordered and so the name stuck.

Twill A weave that forms diagonal lines running to right or left across the fabric.

Ulster A long, loose overcoat made of rough material invented in the 1870s and with a cape covering the shoulders. Referenced in many Sherlock Holmes stories.

Velour The French word for velvet. It is a woollen or cotton fabric with a velvet-like pile.

Velvet True velvet is made of silk. Velvet is a tufted fabric with a soft texture. Some people are known to have a phobia about velvet. Looks great on an evening jacket as it reflects the light. Nothing has the colour density of velvet; the blues and blacks are as intense as any Anish Kapoor sculpture.

Velveteen This is the poor man's velvet made of cotton.

Vicuña – *ver-cuna* The vicuña is one of two wild South American camelids, a relative of the llama, which live in the high alpine areas of the Andes. Vicuñas produce small amounts of extremely fine wool because the animal can only be shorn once every three years. This is one of the most expensive fabrics in existence.

Voile A thin, lightweight woven fabric usually made of cotton or cotton blends including linen or polyester. The term comes from French and means "veil".

Warp The vertical north/south yarn of the weave in fabric. Warp means "that which is thrown across".

Weave The in-and-out interlacing of yarns to produce a piece of fabric.

Weft The weft is the horizontal, east-to-west yarn of the weave of fabric. The weft is threaded through the warp using a shuttle.

Wellington Worn and popularized by Arthur Wellesley, 1st Duke of Wellington, it was originally produced in calfskin, but today is traditionally made in waterproof rubber. Hunter make the classic British Wellington boots.

Welt The bordering of an edge or pocket, which shapes and strengthens it. Can also mean the strip of leather, rubber or plastic, which attaches the sole to the upper in shoemaking.

Windowpane Check A check formed by coloured lines crossing each other to cause square, window-shaped patterning.

Windsor Knot A method of tying a necktie, which results in a thick, wider knot. The tie is double-tied to make it bulkier. There is also a half-Windsor knot, which is not as wide.

Winklepicker A type of shoe with an exaggerated pointed toe. Popular in the 1950s and 1960s, the style resembles French poulaines from the fifteenth century.

Woad A plant that gives a deep blue pigment when used in dyeing. The first-century queen of Britain's Iceni tribe, Boudicca, used woad as a war paint.

Worsted Yarn that has been combed to make it smoother, drawing the fibres into parallel positions. The name derives from the village of Worstead in Norfolk, England. Along with North Walsham and Aylsham, this village became a centre for the manufacture of yarn and cloth after weavers from Flanders arrived in the twelfth century.

Wyncol Wyncol D711 is a virtually wind- and waterproof fabric that is exclusive to the British luxury brand Aquascutum. It was chosen by Edmund Hillary and his team during their first ascent of Mount Everest in 1953. The densely woven cotton and nylon poplin is incredibly lightweight and virtually tear-proof. Aquascutum have re-launched Wyncol D711 in various men's waterproof coats ranging from a classic trench to a coat that can be zipped to form a rucksack.

Yarn The strand of spun fibres used to weave or knit fabric.

Yoke The part of a shirt that stretches over the shoulders, usually made out of a doubled piece of fabric.

Zip A device that temporarily joins two pieces of fabrics. The B. F. Goodrich Company coined the name "zipper" in 1923 for the line of rubber overshoes that it made using the fastener. Slowly the name came to be associated with the fastener itself, and eventually acquired generic status.

Zoot suit An exaggerated suit with high-waisted, wide-legged, tight-cuffed, pegged trousers and a long coat with wide lapels and wide padded shoulders. This style of clothing was popularized by African-American and West Indian men during the late 1930s and 1940s.

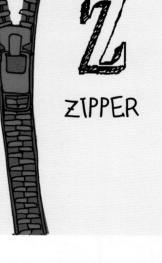

ZIPPER

STOCKISTS & SUPPLIERS

Below are listed the many of the manufacturers, retailers and brands mentioned throughout the book, as well as a number of quintessentially British institutions that have helped to define menswear fashion today.

FASHION

A Bathing Ape
www.bape.com
A Japanese clothing company specializing in artwork-styled streetwear.

American Apparel
http://store.americanapparel.co.uk
Basics such as T-shirts and vests ethically made in the USA.

ASOS
www.asos.com
"As Seen On Screen" sells pretty much everything a young man might need from high-street to designer. ASOS is a great supporter of young designers and brands.

Baracuta
www.baracuta-g9.com
Home of the original Harrington jacket born in England in 1937 and "as worn by Steve McQueen, Elvis and Sinatra".

Barbour
www.barbour.com
Authentic British country and lifestyle clothing brand, known in particular for its hardwearing waxed-cotton jackets.

Bates Hatmakers
A fixture of London's Jermyn Street since 1902, this hatmaker produces traditional British headgear – from top hats to panamas.

Belstaff
www.belstaff.com
Formed in 1924, this British brand with a phoenix logo is world famous for its motor-cycle jackets, boots, and associated products.

Beyond Retro
www.beyondretro.com
For on-trend vintage menswear, such as 1970s cardies, Western plaid shirts and accessories.

Brooks Brothers
www.brooksbrothers.com
Established 1818, Brooks Brothers is the America's oldest clothing retailer introducing the first ready-to-wear suits to the nation. The company has become synonymous with the "Ivy League" look.

Burberry
www.burberry.com
Wearable Englishness, Burberry is the powerhouse of British fashion. Burberry Brit is the younger, sportier range.

Cheap Monday
www.cheapmonday.com
Swedish company famous for its skinny jeans styles and idiosyncratic designs, which also includes sneakers and shirts.

Cherry Blossom
www.cherryblossom.co.uk
Leading brand of shoe-care products.

Christies
www.christies.com/livebidding
Premium auction house selling vintage jewellery and accessories.

Christys' Hatmakers
www.christys-hats.com
Founded in 1773, Christys claims to be the only hatmaker in the world still using 200-year-old traditions of manufacture.

Church's
www.church-footwear.com
Makers of superb quality handmade leather shoes. Each pair takes 8 to 10 weeks to manufacture.

Dior Homme
www.diorhomme.com
The online boutique for Christian Dior menswear, including ready-to-wear, shoes, leather goods, watches, ties, belts and eyewear.

D.S. Dundee
www.dsdundee.com
Luxury modern tweeds inspired by Scottish textile history, based in East London.

E Tautz
www.etautz.com
Founded in 1867 in London's West End and catering to Europe's sporting and military elite as well as royalty. In the past, E Tautz's

handmade clothing was worn by Winston Churchill, David Niven and Cary Grant.

Fendi
www.fendi.com
This Italian brand's menswear line includes ready-to-wear and accessories.

Gucci
www.gucci.com
High-end tailoring and luxury accessories.

Hackett
www.hackett.com
Designer menswear and accessories brand and home to "Essential British kit".

Henry Herbert Tailors
www.henryherbert.com
Bespoke tailors for shirts and suits with a 24-hour "Savile Row by Scooter" service.

Hermès
www.hermes.com
Parisien luxury. Perfect ready-to-wear, ties, scarves, belts, shoes and other accessories.

Holland & Sherry
www.hollandandsherry.com
Established in 1930 in Bond Street London as woollen merchants, Holland & Sherry supplies prestigious bespoke tailors and luxury brands with the finest cloth.

J Brand Denim
www.jbrandjeans.com
LA-based denim brand known for its fit and understated styles.

Jaegar LeCoultre
www.jaeger-lecoultre.com
Swiss-based high-end luxury watch and clock manufacturers.

James Smith & Sons
www.james-smith.co.uk
British manufacturer of top-quality traditional umbrellas and walking sticks, established in 1830.

John Smedley
www.johnsmedley.com
Fine handcrafted knitwear made from New Zealand merino wool and Sea Island cotton.

Kerry Tayor Auctions
www.kerrytaylorauctions.com
One of the most respected vintage clothing auctioneers, Kerry Taylor sells high-quality vintage online, from her London showroom and through auctions held in association with Sotheby's.

Lou Dalton
www.loudalton.com
With a reputation for "rebellious British sportswear, Lou Dalton was established her menswear collection in 2005.

Louis Vuitton
www.louisvuitton.com
French luxury fashion and leather goods founded in 1854, well known for its LV monogram.

Mackintosh
www.mackintosh-uk.com
Traditional British outerwear, including the oiled-cloth trench coat, quilted jacket and rubberized coat, which is made from its innovative, waterproof "Mackintosh Cloth".

Marc Jacobs
www.marcjacobs.com
Men's ready-to-wear, shoes, fragrance and eyewear under the main couture line or the diffusion Marc by Marc Jacobs line.

Moncler V
www.moncler.it
Designed by Hiroki Nakamura and inspired by the Alpine heritage of Moncler.

Mr Porter
www.mrporter.com
Recently launched under former Esquire and Wallpaper editor Jeremy Langmead, this site is the husband to net-a-porter.com.

My Wardrobe
www.my-wardrobe.com
Designer wear Paul Smith, D&G, broken down into casual, contemporary and classic collections as well as denim, holiday and designer.

Norton & Sons
www.nortonandsons.co.uk
Established 1821, Norton & Sons is one of Savile Row's finest bespoke tailors. The company incorporates brands E Tautz & Sons and J Hoare & Co.

Oliver Peoples Eyewear
www.oliverpeoples.com
Manufacturer of glasses and sunglasses, launched in California in 1986.

One Nine Zero Six
www.oneninezerosix.co.uk
A new label featuring contemporary, casual menswear collection made with the finest English cloth by traditional English manufacturers.

Pantherella
www.pantherella.co.uk
High-quality socks for those who buy for "quality, variety and value for money".

Paul Smith
www.paulsmith.co.uk
British designer of high-quality menswear. In addition to his main line, collections include Paul Smith London, PS by Paul Smith, Paul Smith Jeans and Paul Smith Red Ear.

Prada
www.prada.com
Fun, stylish footwear, bags, wallets, belts, sunglasses and other fashion accessories from this luxury Italian line.

RAKE
www.rakestyle.com
New label aimed at the "international man", the RAKE collection is made of versatile separates constructed using only the finest selection of cloths.

Rokit
www.rokit.co.uk
Vintage clothing and accessories, searchable by era.

Shanghai Tang
www.shanghaitang.com
From their bespoke Imperial Tailoring service to a ready-to-wear line, this Chinese boutique couture company interprets Chinese culture and craftsmanship for a twenty-first-century market. Their Mandarin Collar Society champions a modern version of the traditional mandarin-collared shirt.

Sunspel
www.sunspel.com
Sunspel has been making the finest handmade English underwear, T-shirts and polo shirts since 1860.

Swatch
www.swatch.com
Named after "second watch", Swatch introduced the concept of cheap, fun accessories. As well as the original cult plastic watch, there are now metal, skin, jewellery and diving versions.

Topman
www.topman.com
Top menswear trends hot off the catwalk at affordable prices.

Uniqlo
www.uniqlo.com
Japan's leading retail chain with an international presence selling good-quality, inexpensive basics as well as a suits line, +J, in collaboration with Jil Sander.

Zara
www.zara.com
This Spanish clothing and accessories company has a great range of menswear sold internationally through its stores. Known for its super-quick turn around from catwalk to shop floor, the designs are sleek, versatile and comfortable.

GROOMING

Clinique
www.cliniqueformen.co.uk
Skincare solutions for men
including anti-ageing products.

Roja Dove
www.rojadove.com
Probably the world's most
renowned 'nose', this fragrance
specialist and historian now has
his own range of perfumes.

Jo Hansford
www.johansford.com
Leading hair-colour salon based
in London's Mayfair, plus pedicure
and manicure services.

Murdock London
www.murdocklondon.com
Traditional London barbers with
its own range of products.

NW Smiles
www.nwsmiles.co.uk
State-of-the-art London-based
dental surgery near Baker Street,
offering both general dentistry
and cosmetic dentistry services.

Penhaligon's
www.penhaligons.com
English perfume house founded
in the late 1860s. Their first scent
was Hamman Bouquet in 1872,
and their best-selling is Blenheim
Bouquet, launched in 1902.

Proactiv® skincare
www.proactive.co.uk
Range of skincare products
designed to help clear blemishes
and help prevent future
breakouts.

Shavata Brow Studio
www.shavata.co.uk
Eyebrow shaping plus range
of online products to help you
create the perfect brow.

Strip
www.stripwaxbar.com
Funky London waxing salon.
Recommended treatments include
Lycon's MANifico hot wax and
they also sell post-wax products
such as Lycon's sugar scrubs and
Ingrown-X-it.

The Studio
ww.johnniesapong.com
Johnnie Sapong's innovative,
creative London hub for clients
who want to indulge in one-to-one
private hair appointments.

Truefitt & Hill
www.truefittandhill.co.uk
World's oldest barbershop that
sells great grooming products
online from shaving to bathing.

INDEX

ACKNOWLEDGEMENTS

PICTURE CREDITS

The publishers would like to thank the following sources for their kind permission to reproduce the pictures in this book.

Key, t: top, b: bottom, l: left, r: right, c: centre.

Alamy Images: /Moviestore Collection: 24br

barbaranastacio.com: /Barbara Anastacio: 47, 48, 49l, 49c, 49r, 50l, 51l, 52c, 53

Bridgeman Art Library: /Robert Dighton: 16

Corbis: /Bettmann: 22bl, 35, /Sunset Boulevard: 24l

Getty Images: 19, 20br, 21, 31, 33b, 34, 36, 37, 40, /Ulf Andersen: 41, /Bridgeman Art Library: 20l, /Tim Graham: 39, /Redferns: 30, 32, /Time & Life Pictures: 18, /WireImage: 33t

Marcus Jaye: 46l, 46c, 46r, 50r, 51c, 51r, 54l, 55r, 57

mattiarioli.com: /Mattia Arioli: 69c, 69r
Noëllie Fournier: 44l, 44r, 45, 52l, 52r, 56r, 65l, 66l, 66r, 66

PYMCA: 60r, 68l, /Kjeld Duits/JapaneseStreets: 71l, 71r, /Pat Lyttle/Jstreetstyle: 70, /Phil Oh/Street Peeper: 59, 59l, 59r, 60l, 61, 62l, 62c, 62r, 63, 68r, 69l, 73l, 72, 73r, /Wayne Tippetts: 64, 65r

Rex Features: 22tr, 23, /20th Century Fox/Everett: 27, 28r, /Everett Collection: 25, 38, /ITV: 28l, 29

robinmellor.com: /Robin Mellor: 54r, 55l, 56l

Topfoto.co.uk: 17

Every effort has been made to acknowledge correctly and contact the source and/or copyright holder of each picture and Carlton Books Limited apologizes for any unintentional errors or omissions, which will be corrected in future editions of this book.

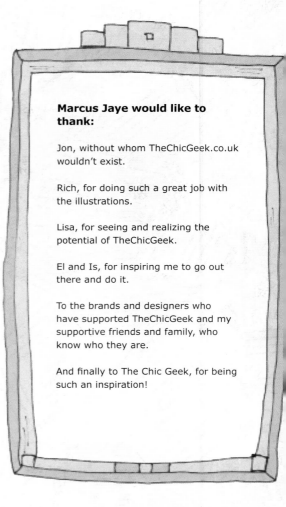

Marcus Jaye would like to thank:

Jon, without whom TheChicGeek.co.uk wouldn't exist.

Rich, for doing such a great job with the illustrations.

Lisa, for seeing and realizing the potential of TheChicGeek.

El and Is, for inspiring me to go out there and do it.

To the brands and designers who have supported TheChicGeek and my supportive friends and family, who know who they are.

And finally to The Chic Geek, for being such an inspiration!